PSYCHE & SUBSTANCE

Essays on Homeopathy in the Light of
Jungian Psychology

PSYCHE and SUBSTANCE

Essays on Homeopathy in the Light of
Jungian Psychology

by

Edward C. Whitmont

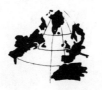

NORTH ATLANTIC BOOKS

ACKNOWLEDGEMENTS

All essays but two in this book were presented at various professional meetings from 1948-1955. They would have remained buried among the files of forgotten reprints had it not been for the insistent urging of Maesimund B. Panos, M.D. To her is owing my foremost indebtedness for the existence of this book. Had it not been for her singlehanded assembling of the various papers and hounding me over all this time to look them over and her finally finding a publisher, I would have waited for a time, perhaps never to arrive, in which a more consistent field theory of psychosomatics could be presented. It is thanks to her efforts that the material is now accessible in this fragmentary form. I hope that it may serve as a help and stimulation to those who care to pioneer the dark borderland where psyche and matter intertwine in the mystery of the dematerialized substance.

I am indebted to Dana Ullman who on his own initiative gathered and began to disseminate this material and to Richard Grossinger who has undertaken the task of publishing it with him.

I also wish to thank *Spring Publications* for permission to reprint "Nature, Symbol, and Imaginal Reality" and Princeton University Press for the quotes of Carl G. Jung.

The Collected Works of C.G. Jung, translated by R.F.C. Hull, Bollingen Series XX. Excerpts reprinted by permission of Princeton University Press.

Special thanks to Barbara T. Blair who transposed footnotes to the *Collected Works* of Carl Jung (Princeton University Press) in six of the articles.

Some of these articles appeared previously in *The Homeopathic Recorder* and the *Journal of the American Institute of Homeopathy.*

PSYCHE AND SUBSTANCE: Essays on Homeopathy in the Light of Jungian Psychology

Copyright 1980 by Edward C. Whitmont   ISBN 0-913028-67-3
Second printing: Copyright 1982 by Edward C. Whitmont   ISBN 0-913028-66-5 (pbk.)

Publishers' Addresses: North Atlantic Books   Homeopathic Educational Services
                        2320 Blake Street   2124 Kittredge Street
                        Berkeley, CA 94704   Berkeley, CA 94704

Cover: David Bullen
Cover Photograph: Planetary Nebula NGC 7293 in Aquarius. 200 inch Hale telescope.

Library of Congress Cataloging in Publication Data

Whitmont, Edward C., 1912-
    Psyche & substance.

    Includes bibliographical references.
    1. Homeopathy—Addresses, essays, lectures.
2. Jung, C. G. (Carl Gustav), 1875-1961.
I. Title.   II. Title: Psyche and substance.
RX78.W5   1983   615.5′32′019   82-22322
ISBN 0-913028-66-5 (pbk.)

CONTENTS

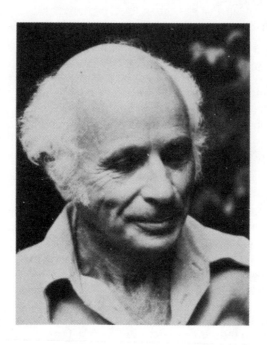

Edward C. Whitmont was graduated from the Vienna University Medical School in 1936 and had early training in Adlerian psychology. In 1937 he studied Rudolf Steiner's work with Karl Konig, later founder of the Camphill Movement. An initial interest in psychosomatics and holistic approaches led him into research in the areas of naturopathy, chiropractic, nutrition, yoga and astrology beginning in 1940. During this time he studied homeopathy with Elizabeth Wright Hubbard and medical dowsing with G. B. Stearns. From 1947 through 1951 he taught homeopathy at the Postgraduate School of the American Foundation for Homeopathy. A concurrent interest in Analytical Psychology led to correspondence and meetings with Carl G. Jung and training in Jungian therapy with various teachers including M. Esther Harding. He is presently in private practice of Analytical Psychology in New York while teaching at the C. G. Jung Training Center, of which he is a founding member and chairman. He is the author of *The Symbolic Quest: Basic Concepts of Analytical Psychology* (Princeton University Press).

INTRODUCTION:
"Aude sapere"

The remedy pictures in this volume, written mostly 25 to 30 years ago, were attempts to explore a new way of thinking which I would call imaginal and analogical as opposed to abstract and causalistic. By and large this mode of thinking has until recently been restricted to the artist's domain. The sober halls of science have been closed to such thinking as they have been closed to a consideration of homeopathy and its implications, practical and theoretical.

Eighteenth and nineteenth century rationalism and positivism, fellow travellers of mercantilism and industrialism, could think only in terms of mechanistic causation and survival usefulness. The idea that form and patterns are a play of nature with no purpose other than their own fulfillment was utterly foreign and unacceptable to them. Yet processes of form, we have discovered in microphysics as well as in Jung's work in depth psychology, underlie the basic dynamics of both matter and psyche. Form implies pattern, analogy and even esthetics. Hence the perception and recognition of analogical forms requires a special sensitivity that is not ordinarily a part of our scientific training. Yet it can prove itself an eminently useful means of unravelling functional interrelations and pointing up directions of energy and manifestations. Over and above mechanical and chemical dynamics, form patterns are expressions of symbolic correlations, correlations of analogy or similarity, of 'as if'. Similarly, nuclear physics uses symbolic images in order to create models of the behavior of ultimate entities not otherwise describable; and depth psychology has discovered that symbolic images and correlations are among the most powerful transmittors of energy, capable of 'moving mountains'.

Imaginal and symbolic thinking is moreover eminently helpful in grasping the constitutional 'remedy pictures' of the homeopathic materia medica. Beyond that it may open our eyes to a new view of existence helping us conceive how psyche and soma, man and earth function as different aspects of one integrated field. As such this view is no longer new today. It is talked about among environmentalists and those interested in humanistic and transpersonal psychology as well as Eastern religions. But in terms of specific application, this viewpoint has not advanced too far beyond a sort of new romanticism, a philosophy of life, which may be important and valuable, but with the exception of some brain research, it has had as yet relatively little influence upon practical scientific work.

Homeopathy, on the other hand, presents us with a veritable treasure house of practical data, utterly confusing at first and mindblowing to traditional scientific thought. If these data were accepted as verifiable they would call for a revision of many basic assumptions in physiology, psychobiology and pathology. Chemistry and mechanics could no longer be considered the fundamental regulators. Form, images — as archetypal, autonomous indeed transcendental patterns prior to and playing with substance, directing the life force and hence biochemistry, physiology and psychology — would prove to be the basic regulators. These autonomous form patterns transcend as well as include what we are in the habit of separating into compartments of within, without, of soul and body, man and nature, of health and pathology, of solid substance and impalpable energy. "Everything transient is but a symbol..." (J.W. Goethe, Faust 2nd part.)

Yet such an imaginal science, willing and capable of thinking in symbolic patterns is barely beginning in our day and was totally absent in Hahnemann's time. Hence the theoretical foundations of homeopathy could not and 'must not' be true according to orthodox scientists. They thought this way not because it does not work, but because it 'could not possibly work' on a priori grounds of biased conviction. Medical and biological scientists consequently refused to investigate the claims of homeopathy by clinical trial. Those few who individually tried became convinced homeopaths.

One is reminded of the time of Galileo, Copernicus and Kepler when the idea or possibility of the earth rather than the sun being the moving body was rejected out of hand as heretical. Galileo's clerical contemporaries refused to even look into a telescope to verify the moons of Jupiter he claimed to have discovered. Scriptural tradition made no reference to Jovian moons, therefore, they could not, must not exist. The human mind tends to cling to established views as to a religion which promises security of order as over and against chaos. Any challenge to habitual views is a threat to this sense of religious security. This is as true in our 'enlightened, rational' day as it was in past 'dark' centuries. Only the name of the infallible dogma has changed. 'Holy church teaches' has become 'Science teaches.' And religions and existential convictions change but slowly.

Nuclear physicists have discovered that in the realm of the subatomic, nature behaves in ways entirely different from what we believe to perceive with the naked eye and our ordinary common sense. That which we call visible matter is but a symbolic perception 'as if' it were a condensation of something unknown, perhaps unknowable, but at best describable and operative in terms of images such as the model of an atom or a psychic stratum. It is 'Formation, Transformation, Eternal mind's Eternal recreation.' (Goethe, Faust part 2.) Yet we continue to deal with everyday reality as if image and psychic dynamics were irrelevant and separate from 'material' events which are still considered largely chance determined.

8

In our time of transition there is by way of compensation the opposite tendency of confusing holism with psychologism, of viewing all pathology as secondary to psychological attitudes. The old Cartesian dichotomy is still prevalent in such an approach but with reversed denominators. The body is here treated as an epiphenomenon of the mind rather than as formerly the other way around. Now a 'right' attitude of mind is held to be the exclusive determinant in curing or preventing illness by avoiding stress and tension. While it is certainly true that a hopeless or pessimistic outlook on life, repressed psychological conflicts and tensions do result in organic pathology and that positive imaging helps in restoring as well as maintaining health, it is equally true that no one alive can wholly avoid tension, stress, conflict, repressions, depression and disappointment. Indeed psychological complexes and crises are building stones of personality. Frustration and repression are the unavoidable conditions of egobuilding no less than approval, success, satisfaction and joy. The capacity to become ill seems to be built into the ground plan of human nature regardless of mental efforts to the contrary. Moreover, we are not merely free floating minds but minds embodied. A genuinely holistic viewpoint cannot but see the body as the visibility of the mind and the mind as the expression of the particular individual self's way of embodiment. Just as our psyches are open to and indeed participate in the energy patterns that surround us, so our bodies interact with substance and are parts of earth processes and nature. And nature is not only kind and lifesupporting; it is also destructive and terrible. Natural living does not guarantee health. Indeed a perfectly natural way of living would amount to a return to savagery. Primitive man also knew illness. Civilization undoubtedly produces its own pathology but natural primitiveness does also. Whichever way we turn we cannot avoid crisis, pain and disease. The tendency to illness appears to be an aspect of the earth dynamic, as is healing. They are the two sides of the same coin. "That which wounded shall heal" is the oldest known formulation of the similia similibus curentur,* wisdom of the unconscious or of the gods and is ascribed to the Delphic oracle in reply to the injury of Telephos. (Telephos means the far shining light.)

The evidence of the homeopathic provings† and of the efficacy of the simillimum selected from the specific symptom totality demonstrates the fact that for every possibility of personality as well as organismic

*Like may be cured by like, known as The Law of Similars in homeopathy.
†For the definition of provings and description of their methodology, see the article entitled "Toward a Basic Law of Psychic and Somatic Interrelationship."

pattern, hence for every possibility of illness pattern there is also a substance pattern 'out there' which minutely duplicates it. The provings show that every existing substance contains or embodies a disordering potential of human existence that can be activated by the process of potentisation, a desubstantialisation which turns even the so-called 'inert' substances into potent agents. The proving disorder is brought about by insistent repetition or simple overdosing of what in a single dose would heal. The proving disorder demonstrates the effect of disbalance, here deliberately produced, spontaneous in natural illness. Discontinuance of the disbalancing proving results in restoration of balance. (Unless the restorative power has been overwhelmed by injudicious use; then we speak of poisoning.)

Medieval alchemists held man to be a microcosmic replica of the macrocosmos of nature. Hence Paracelsus felt that diseases should be classified as diseases of lead, silver, gold, Saturn, moon, sun or some other substance according to the cosmic patterns that correspond to and activate them. This contention is experimentally and clinically born out by homeopathy. Every disturbance of health, be it organic or merely functional, is a 'cry for the remedy' or as Hering put it, a cry for the process that is its macrocosmic form analogon and that can restore balance when brought into confrontatin with the disease process. When the outer and the inner process are brought into confrontation, they seem to cancel each other. Yet it is more than a cancelling: underactivity is stimulated, overactivity is calmed. Imbalance is illness, confrontation restores balance and heals.

Yet that which eventually can heal can also make us ill. And only that which can make us ill can also heal. To be alive means to remain exposed to the tidal swing of balance-disbalance and to experience and confront both.

No safe a priori middle ideal exists that would insure permanent normalcy. The very attempt to cling to such a 'safe' riskless path that avoids experimentation and discovery creates its own compensatory pathology of unlived life and rigidity. We have learned that much from depth psychology, and the pathology of retirement seems to confirm it. Going out of one's way to avoid trouble only calls it forth in another form. 'Expect poison from stagnant waters', warned Blake.

Psychologically, growth of personality occurs through crisis and confrontation with archetypal, namely specifically typical human patterns, situations or problems such as dependence, separation, togetherness, competition, aggression, love; the complexes of father, mother, child, the hero, or of evil to name but a few. Psychopathology ensues when the challenges of these patterns are not adequately met with awareness. Then they may threaten to overwhelm us. Conscious confrontation, deliberate working through with full emotional and bodily experiencing and symbolic realisation as in psychodrama or in encounter situations protects us from the compulsion of destructive "acting out", from being victimized by our complexes. The potentially destructive impulses are 'attenuated' through deliberate confrontation techniques; and through symbolic 'as if' experiences a dimension of meaning, a quasi-spiritual core is activated which leads to a new balance between ego and drives.

It is an amazing testimony to the unity of cosmic existence that the analogous dynamic is also to be found on the biological and organic level in temperamental, constitutional and 'acute' adaptive imbalances in the form of illnesses which call for their archetypal counterpattern to be confronted through the simillimum in its attenuated 'symbolic' potency or dynamic essence.

Health and illness are but variants of the same life dynamic, balanced or imbalanced, integrated or disintegrating, differentiated or undifferentiated expressions of archetypal form patterns.

Since the life process is a constant play of form fluidly groping, experimenting with new possibilities and variants of differentiation, balance is ever and again shifted by risking imbalance. Normalcy and abnormalcy, illness and health are the ways, seemingly, by which life reaches for ever finer differentiation. And spirit and life pertain to the 'inwardness', as Teilhard de Chardin called it, of substance, animate or inanimate, 'out there' no less than within ourselves. Yet inward and outward, within and without are at best symbolic images. They apply concepts of space to dimensions of reality that are beyond space and time and comprehension. Through our concrete life and with the help of imaginal capacities we need constantly to encounter, confront and integrate them symbolically and experimentally.

In concluding I feel I must sound a warning from the angle of practical homeopathic prescribing. The remedy-personality pictures here attempted provide only one of many possible approaches to the Materia Medica study. I would call it a bird's eye view of what otherwise can get lost in the maze of details. Yet this bird's eye view may omit details of decisive importance in a given situation. The overview can help us see a context of meaning in the details which otherwise must be memorised mechanically; indeed it may sometimes lead to an accurate prescription by itself particularly in chronic, constitutional states.

However, due to constantly overlapping constitutional similarities the step from the simile to the simillium which alone will do the trick, requires careful restudy of modalities and particulars which only repertorial and materia medica comparison can provide.

Part I
AN OVERVIEW

THE PRACTICE OF HOMEOPATHY

I shall first try to answer a question which I have been asked repeatedly and which I have sometimes asked myself. Why is there such a lack of familiarity with, and acceptance of, Homeopathy by so many physicians? I believe there is a basic reason for this which should not be underestimated. The difficulty which at the outset blocks the understanding of Homeopathy lies in the fact that its approach is quite fundamentally at variance with the prevailing approach to science — and mark, I said *approach to science;* I did not say *scientific approach* — namely that method generally adopted throughout the past hundred years. Homeopathy's approach is finalistic and phenomenalistic rather than causalistic. Homeopathy does not evaluate the situation — an illness, for instance — from the standpoint of "what is the causative agent," which is the standard procedure of modern medicine. It does not ask what infection, what abnormal chemistry, what change in structure, and so forth, lies at the bottom of the disease and obviously, therefore, has to be removed, but it addresses itself to what we may call the phenomenon of constitutional totality. It considers the *wholeness* of the phenomenon in *descriptive* rather than causalistic terms.

Now it would seem that what I have said, almost by definition and by the condemnation of my own words, would brand Homeopathy as unscientific, for is it not obvious that one must seek out the cause of anything wrong and then remove it? Indeed, Homeopathy has been called unscientific for the exact reason that it declined to proceed in that manner, and many who have tried to grapple with it have found its approach rather peculiar.

Here I shall present the testimony of a modern scientist — Robert Oppenheimer of the Institude for Advanced Study at Princeton — quoting from a speech that he gave in March 1956 to an assembled group of psychologists:

> I would like to say something about what physics has to give back to common sense that it seemed to have lost from it . . . because it seems to me that the worst of all possible misunderstandings would be that psychology be influenced to model itself after a physics which is not there any more, which has been quite outdated.
>
> We inherited at the beginning of this century a notion of the physical world as a causal one in which every event could be accounted for if we were ingenious, a world characterized by number, where everything interesting could be measured and quantified, a determinist world, a world in which there

was no room for individuality in which the object of study was simply there and how you studied it did not affect the object...

This extremely rigid picture left out a great deal of common sense...

We have five things which we have got back into physics ...with complete objectivity in the sense that we understand each other with a complete lack of ambiguity and with perfectly phenomenal technical success.

One of them is...that the physical world is not completely determinate. There are predictions you can make about it but they are statistical; and any event has in it the nature of a surprise, of the miracle, of something that you could not figure out. Physics is predictable but within limits; its world is ordered but not completely causal.

...Classical science was differential. Anything that went on could be broken into finer elements and analyzed so... Every pair of observations taking the form "we know this, we then predict that" is a global thing; it cannot be broken down.

Finally every atomic event is individual. It is not in its essentials reproducible. *Analogy in Sciences,* Robert Oppenheimer, Institute for Advanced Study. *The American Psychologist, March 1956).*

Translated into plain English all of this means that in modern physics we have come to realize that phenomena cannot always be explained in terms of a cause and effect chain in which a cause leads to a predictable effect, but that they have to be understood in an entirely different sense as quasi-individualistic parts of a grand total of an encompassing pattern. An example of this is what is defined as an energy field. Within the field pattern the various effects are not causally dependent upon each other; thus they can be predicted in their arrangement only statistically; and a field is *defined* not as it "is" this or that but only indirectly — that is, descriptively — through the patterns and forms of matter that manifest its influence. It is basic for our modern artifices. We cannot say what it is — we do not know. We can only say how it behaves. We do this by describing a number of phenomena and facts which make up a patterned grand total — a picture. And this is precisely the way in which the homeopath goes about assaying what he deals with in illness. He arranges, assays, collects, a picture. We speak and think in terms of *remedy pictures.* We assay that expression of an energy field of the illness, unknown per se, but found and manifesting itself in the way it arranges the symptoms — or shall we say, the expressions of the disturbed physiologic functioning — and we compare this field effect, this grand total image, with a similar field effect which has been observed by exposing the organism to the energy field of the drug. Thereby we establish the exact drug action and drug energy in the form of a drug image. The therapeutic thinking in terms of such a phenomenologically descriptive field which thereby addresses itself, not to the cause and effect chain, but to the grand constitutional total manifested in the field phenomenon, leads to what we call constitutional prescribing. In practical terms it means that Homeopathy never deals with an overt disease manifestation — with an infection, shall we say — but with that disturbance which enables the infection to take hold, *contains* it, as it were, as a partial element. It does not deal with an effect of changed chemistry, but with that energy, that ordering element, which permits this change of chemistry to occur.

Perhaps now you see that this difference of approach has two very practical aspects, 1) in terms of *how we go about it;* and 2) *what we bring about.* The constitutional totality method differs from usual medicine in the way it sets about selecting the drug, and in what it expects the drug to bring about. It differs in the same fashion, if I may use an analogy, as an attempt to ward of smallpox, *in olden* times, by hanging up cloths soaked with disinfectant or burning incense, differs from modern immunization by vaccination. In saying this I am neither advocating nor rejecting vaccination. I merely use the analogy in order to describe an approach that mobilizes the defense forces, the immunizing forces, of the organism itself rather than one that attempts to stop an "invasion" directly. This immunizing defensive ability seems to be a general phenomenon and by far exceeds what is at present known to us from the limited field of immunology, which constitutes, after all, a very limited application of the homeopathic or isopathic principle.

This does not mean, however, that because the symptoms of the disturbed condition are used in this descriptive fashion to arrive at a medicine, Homeopathy treats symptoms. This is as incorrect as it would be to say, for instance, that the geiger counter indicates noises. The geiger counter merely *uses* a noise phenomenon — a clicking — to indicate the presence of radiation not directly perceptible. Similarly, the symptoms are used to indicate the presence of an otherwise imperceptible energy disturbance, comparable to the radiation in the above example.

Now what symptoms does Homeopathy use? It uses those symptoms that are indicative of the disturbed energy field, namely, of the individual physiological reaction or expression of reaction. In other words, it selects those symptoms — or shall we say it directs itself according to those symptoms — that make the individual condition unique, different from any other, and at the same time are most expressive of the encompassing wholeness of the individual under observation. Those symptoms are what we call *general* symptoms — symptoms that affect the *whole* individual, not only parts; mental symptoms, meaning symptoms expressive of the way the *personality* reacts; the strange, rare and peculiar symptoms such as are indicative of this particular individual's response; and also symptoms that are strange, rare and peculiar inasmuch as they do not logically fit into the expected clinical picture. For instance, when someone with an acute fever is very hungry and not thirsty. This is a peculiar symptom because in fever ordinarily one is thirsty and has no appetite, so that it is something rather unusual when a person is not thirsty but is hungry. It is typical of an individual energy field arrangement.

Now in these few words we have in a nutshell what Homeopathy really stands for. *That* is Homeopathy. Homeopathy is *not* the prescribing of small doses. The question of dosage is incidental, purely pragmatic. It has nothing to do with the principal issue of Homeopathy, apart from the fact that Homeopathy does not actually prescribe *small doses* but potentized medicines — substances altered in respect to their qualitative, not quantitive, state.

In order to make this as concrete as possible I will give you an example of homeopathic prescribing. We will consider the case history of a patient seen for what is known as paroxysmal tachycardia. This is a state where there are attacks of extremely rapid heartbeat, a pulse rate up to 150 or even faster, and these were the complaints for which this patient sought medical advice.

The clinical workup showed that he was also suffering from valvular insufficiency, probably of rheumatic origin. However, the attacks themselves had come only relatively recently and had no obvious connection with the pre-existing valvular condition. He had been taking quinidin for a long time with fairly satisfactory success but he wanted to see if he could not get rid of it permanently. In addition to the main complaints he had a history of intestinal spasticity, ringing in the ears and right-side sacro-iliac disturbances. The laboratory report did not produce anything else of interest except for the electrocardiogram, which more or less confirmed the cardiac diagnosis. So far this is a complete clinical picture which would indicate the drugs which had been prescribed — digitalis or quinidin. He had them.

Now what does the homeopath do about this? The homeopath would answer: "Nothing, because I have not the case yet. With that history I know nothing whatsoever about the patient. In practical terms, it is a completely meaningless situation and I have not the faintest idea what drug he needs because the most important information has not yet been made available." What is this missing information? We will consult my case sheet.

I asked him first: "Tell me everything that bothers you — everything whatsoever, even the slightest and most irrelevant complaint, regardless of whether it has anything to do with your main trouble." So he told me that sometimes his vision is blurred. Then he mentioned the rumblings in the abdomen and a tendency to loose stools; he said that he has ringing in the ears; he gets tired; and he has sacro-iliac trouble on the right side. There is also a feeling of tenderness in the abdomen — an X-ray fifteen years ago showed dropped intestines. He said also that when he is either tense, sits a great deal and doesn't move around, his troubles begin. So I said to him: "It's a bit better, but still I know nothing about you." I asked further and this is what I elicited.

He used to be very fond of sweets — has a craving for sweets; would pick up any piece of candy he could find. Funny, is it not? And how apparently silly and irrelevant! He feels better when he moves around; is very logy after sitting but gets relief if he moves around vigorously. The buzzing sound in the ears is worse on the right side; I checked again on his sacro-iliac trouble — was that also on the right side? It was. So I asked him: "Are most of your troubles on the right side?" Well no, he didn't think so. "What about your abdominal troubles," I asked? Oh, yes, also on the right! I wrote down "right-sided." Then upon questioning he remembered that much more often than not his attacks come on in the late afternoon. Which did not satisfy me — "What *is* the late afternoon — three, four, five, six, seven o'clock?" Well, it is from four o'clock on. Then, he is happier when he is warm, gets chilled easily, but also feels better in the open air. He does not like to have his abdomen pressed. When I first asked him about this, he said no, he didn't mind. Then I looked at his pants — he was wearing them way down low. I asked him why, and he said that he likes to wear his belt over the bones. Again, why does he like this? And he told me that he didn't like the pressure. I had never seen him with a hat. Why? He did not own a hat. Why not? Well, he did not like hats — did not like the pressure around his head.

After that I was satisfied. I had my remedy. How? Let me give you an example of a drug picture (you remember I spoke of a picture) as it appears when it is observed and tested after we give it to a healthy person. I described the drug I used in this case in the following terms when I was teaching at the Postgraduate School of Homeopathy. The people who are most likely to need it are those who labor intellectually. They are intellectuals of a weak physical constitution. They are people who may lack assurance; who are introverted; with a tendency to brooding; full of fears, anticipation, looking prematurely old, with furrowed faces; who are at the same time afraid of and averse to being alone but equally averse to having company around. In fact, they are happiest when they know someone is in the next room. They are irascible, quite irritable; and relapse easily into their brooding state.

19

They live entirely in the head. They have low powers of resistance to infection, are likely to be dark-complexioned, turn gray early, and do not like to be fenced in either physically or mentally — this last indicated by the reaction to the pressure of clothes, to anything tight around them. Usually their complaints are on the right side of the organism, including a propensity to liver disturbances. Easily chilled, they nevertheless cannot stand heat, are better in the open air and better from motion. Usually their troubles are worse in the late afternoon, between four and eight. One also finds them generally domineering, taciturn, averse to talking, greedy, miserly, and easily moved emotionally; very conservative, prone to suffer from wounded pride, hypochondriacal, over-disputative, oversensitive to noise, craving sweets, with a tendency to flatulence, worse from cold drinks.

Perhaps I need not go into more details after this characterization. One would only add that they are very subject to chronic diseases. Mind you, this is the overall, the most important part of the remedy selection, because whether the patient develops this condition or that one — let us say a coryza or a sore throat or a hepatitis or a pneumonia — is less important. For these types, whenever this remedy is indicated, one finds a right sidedness — a right-sided tonsil condition, right-sided pains, a liver affection, etc. It will be indicated in cases of pneumonia, and in all sorts of intestinal trouble. But the diagnosis is of secondary importance, because whenever the grand total of its characteristic symptoms as described above is present, whatever happens to be the anatomical state or the name of the clinical disease, *Lycopodium,* which is the remedy indicated, will cure if there is no irreversible pathology. Therefore, to know that this is a case of paroxysmal tachycardia helps me as little as to know that he has a tonsillitis or a pneumonia. What I needed to know was how he reacted in terms of those apparently silly, irrelevant peculiarities which Homeopathy calls constitutional symptoms. Then I will give the remedy whether it happens to be tonsillitis or a boil on the back of his neck. This, of course, does not mean that I am not interested in whether or not he has pneumonia, but the fact that a certain clinical picture is present is significant only in that certain drugs have a greater propensity than others to affect certain organs or organ groups. For remedy selection, the exact nature of the condition may be of differential diagnostic importance.

Perhaps I should remind you that in the ordinary pharmacopoeia *Lycopodium* is classed as an inert substance, therapeutically ineffective. By old-time pharmacists it was used as a powder to coat pills – a completely harmless, inert agent. And inert it is. If you take a small dose of it, it will be inert; if you take less *Lycopodium,* it will still be inert; if you take a smaller dose, it will be "inerter"; and if you take still less, it will be "inerterer"! If you decide, as has been ironically suggested, to put a "drop of it into the Hudson," it will do nothing. Because this has nothing to do with Homeopathy. Homeopathy does something entirely different. Instead of making it into "less," it somehow, by a specific process of surface dispersion, increases its energetic charge. We deal here with phenomena not yet sufficiently well understood, theoretically belonging to some sort of electrical field, possibly something akin to surface forces. What matters is that in terms of quantity it is not *less* of something — not less *Lycopodium* — but in energetic terms *more surface effect,* or perhaps an ionizing effect. All I can say is that it is analogous to this group of phenomena with which we are familiar.

I do not know whether further examples are needed. Perhaps another one, in the care of acute conditions, might be simpler. This was a patient hospitalized with pleuro-pneumonia — also on the right side. Here the picture was a bit confused. I do not recall how it started, but when I saw her she had begun under achromycin for two weeks, and was still continuing to fever — apparently an antibiotic-resistant type of pneumonia, since she had had a number of antibiotics before. The peculiar symptoms were that she wanted to lie absolutely still; her pains were of the "stitching" kind; she was very thirsty and she felt better when lying on the painful side.

Now these three symptoms, these peculiarities, point towards a certain drug — *Bryonia.* It was given, and it had no effect. This shows the sort of problems we may run into — what the technical aspects of the situation are. Here we have a case in which the obvious, apparently indicated, remedy did not work. However, we are not yet through. This drug was selected entirely on the basis of the symptoms pertaining to the *immediate illness.* Which means that the symptoms I described — pain on the right side, improvement from pressure, etc., were those of the acute response to the pneumonia. They were not really generalities in the wider constitutional sense. They were still, in a way, the symptoms of the acute disease and not of the individual, and while sometimes that is sufficient, often it is not. So now, practically speaking, what is the *individual?* Well, this individual was a person of a generally pale, waxy, anemic appearance, extremely nervous and hypersensitive. She jumped at every noise — she would jump if someone looked or squinted at her, if she thought they didn't look pleasantly at her. And the symptoms had been changing a great deal during the last two weeks. She did not want meat, she wanted cold milk all the time — always had. Her general desire was for open air and yet she felt chilly on uncovering; and she always had a tendency, now increased, to perspire at night. This new picture, as you see, leaves the pneumonia picture completely behind. It gives us something different. It adds up to a picture of a constitutional peculiarity which is to be found in the provings of

21

Tuberculin, and a dose of that remedy did, in forty-eight hours, what the preceding two weeks of antibiotics — and Homeopathy — did not. It is worth noting that in our listing of the *Tuberculin* indications — the *Tuberculin* symptoms — we find: "failure to respond to the seemingly well-indicated remedy." Thus her lack of response to what we would call the acute remedy was in itself a constitutional sign pointing to another definite drug.

In conclusion, I will offer you one other example. This is a case of a manic-depressive psychosis. Should there be any doubt about this, the date I have here of the first interview is May 2, 1945, which means that the case has been followed and observed for over thirteen years. At the time the patient was first seen she had just been dismissed from a state hospital after her third or fourth sojourn there. The manic attacks occurred at intervals of about every eight or ten months. This state, you know, is one in which the patients go from deep depressions into states of exhilaration and even violence. She had had to be hospitalized because she became quite threatening to her family, and the procedure had to be repeated quite regularly for three or four years. She would be hospitalized; then dismissed with remission of her symptoms; then within a short time there would be evidence that she would need hospitalization again. This time the question arose whether this endless cycle could be stopped.

This is the way I took the case. First she was asked to tell me everything that bothered her. She said she has pains and aches over all the body all the time. She has throbbing headaches at the base of the head. She is dizzy on standing, has sciatica, arthritis of the spine and sometimes interference with vision — blurring. When she has a mental disturbance, she has pleasant thoughts about world peace. When in that state she cannot sleep, but keeps walking and talking. I saw her at such a time. Walk she did — and also, talk she did. In addition, she says her joints are getting stiff, she feels a cracking in the back of the spine; her neck pains when she begins to move it; and there is numbness of the hands. The sockets of the eyes feel very tender. She has eructations, sour taste and heartburn, a tendency to constipation; and a very poor appetite with an aversion to coffee. There is aversion to sex relations; aversion to strong light; she is better indoors; and she is very impatient. Her menses are weak and short. She feels worse before the menstruation and is very depressed before and during menstruation. She is sensitive to touch — hates it if someone touches her. She has a constricting sensation in her throat, is intolerant of anything tight around the waist, and is afraid of and averse to taking a bath. She sleeps deeply, and cries easily, particularly about beautiful things. She has an aversion to company, has indefinite fears and worries, as though something may happen, a poor memory; and a feeling of frustration all over. She is very chilly, sometimes with sensations as if she had chills running up and down the spine, and she catches cold very frequently. She is worse in a damp, cold place. She has a great dislike of milk, but likes sweets and has a desire for salty food.

Now let us see how the case worked out. I used the symptoms: Aversion to coffee; depression; sadness before the menses; menstruation scanty; worse from touch; lack of vital heat; deep sleep; desire for sweets; desire for salty things. Here I used what is called the *repertory* method. We have a book—*the* book, which lists for every symptom observed in the proving, all the remedies that show it. So that when we have a very puzzling case, we can play those symptoms against each other and see what drugs have all of them. Whereas the first symptom — aversion to coffee—is found in about fifty or sixty different drugs, after running through all of the symptoms, only two drugs stood out. One was lime — carbonate of lime — and the other was sodium chloride — table salt. Like *Lycopodium,* table salt is classed as an inert substance. Unless of course it is subjected to that same peculiar process as the other — that is, the repeated rhythmical process of dispersion, thus increasing its surface energy. Now we still have the question — which of the two drugs? So I looked carefully at the patient. She was rather small of stature, very fat, roundish, plump, dry skin, fair complexion. This is how we describe the picture of *Calcarea Carbonica;* this is the type. The *Natrum Muriaticum* type is rather thin, scrawny, very active and tense—not at all like the rather phlegmatic *Calcarea Carbonica.* *Calcarea Carbonica* was the remedy here and it was given at varying intervals. It is now thirteen years since she first had it and there has not been a single hospitalization. This patient is a music teacher and is working in the West. She writes and reports occasionally, and I last saw her a year ago when she was in New York. To all intents and purposes she is well — neither a manic nor a depressive — though I wouldn't say that she doesn't talk much! I used potencies from the 200th up, and there has not been any intervening psychosis although there was one light spell six months after starting treatment for which she was almost hospitalized.

Of course this could be pure coincidence. But thirteen years is a pretty good period for observation.

TOWARDS A BASIC LAW OF PSYCHIC
AND SOMATIC INTERRELATIONSHIP

> Were not the eye to sun akin
> The sun we never could behold
> Filled not a God's strength us within
> How could the divine hold us enthralled?
>
> Goethe: Sprüche 130

Independently of each other, medicine and psychology have accumulated a considerable amount of information in their particular fields. Much less progress has been made, on the other hand, towards an understanding of how these two fields could be systematically correlated. The diagnosis of a disorder as psychosomatic, still implies the absence of "real" organic disease; that psychological difficulties might have very "real" physical manifestations is seldom considered seriously. The general trend of medical thought is still strictly dualistic; psychic and somatic happenings are treated as mutually exclusive rather than inclusive.

Even where there is an inclination to look for a oneness in the dual expressions there is no understanding, as yet, as to where and at what level a synthesis can be found and how one could advance from general philosophical speculations to a really scientific method. A truly scientific method must be able to explain the correlation of specific physio-pathologic and psychologic facts in each given instance; in addition it must enable us to predict facts and connections not yet actually discovered. Instead of this we have only empty words of psychosomatic or psychophysical parallelism which utterly fail to render any specific help or information when put to the practical test.

In attempting to formulate the modest beginnings of such a theory, the bare experimental and clinical evidence, so far known, is made the starting point for finding the basic laws into which those facts can be fitted.

In doing so, we must be aware, however, that the mode of thinking which is applicable to mechanic and inorganic functioning is not in the same way adequate to do full justice to the expressions of life. Life evolves not, as it were, in straight progressions but has a peculiar, often apparently self contradictory forward and backward motion of polar oppositions, complementary expressions and circles.

Complementation, of two entities means that only both together represent the whole; the same road is travelled, the same ends are accomplished by what, on the surface, may appear as different or even opposite means and ways.

Whereas any evolutionary goal is never considered for the physical organization, modern analytical psychology has shown that psychic events, even in their pathologic manifestation as neuroses, represent definite stepping stones in an evolutionary pattern which strives towards the fulfillment of a potentially inherent ideal personality, a wholeness growing out of the resolution and integration of opposing elements.[1]

Once such an evolution is recognized for the psychic half, its physical counterpart, if truly complementary, must necessarily be subject to a corresponding, complementary evolution. Our task would seem to lie in being able successfully to demonstrate somatic events as part of a correlated psychosomatic total evolution, and in finding the dynamic categories or laws which represent the common elements of these complementary psychic and physical evolutions. In short, we are looking for a "generalized field theory" of psychosomatics.

In order to avoid mere speculative theories we must base our hypothesis upon observable or, still better, upon experimental material which would encompass psychic as well as somatic phenomena. Since the psyche of the animal differs fundamentally from the human one, only experiments with human beings can render reliable information for this purpose.

The only such large-scale controlled psychosomatic experiments upon human beings are to be found in the so-called homeopathic "provings". The evidence of psychosomatic interaction gathered from these experimental drug provings may serve as the starting point for our investigation.

In these experiments human "provers", namely people of average health, take repeated doses of drugs until subjective or objective symptoms of a disturbance appear. Those symptoms which are observed with a certain regularity in the majority of people, proving a given drug, are considered to express the characteristic pathogenetic effect of this drug. When, in turn, the symptom complex of any case of spontaneous illness is compared with the artificial symptoms complexes produced by drugs, there will always be found a resemblance, often extraordinarily close, between the disease picture and the picture of the effects of some drug on healthy persons. The drug whose own symptomatology presents the clearest and closest resemblance to the symptom complex of the sick person has clinically been found to be the most successful drug for the treatment of this condition. (Hahnemann's Law of Similars: "Likes should be treated with likes.")

A detailed study of the Homeopathic Materia Medica, which is compiled by collecting these artificial drug pictures and clinical corroborations shows that every such drug effect is characterized by specific alterations of the *total personality,* namely by emotional and mental changes which arise in addition to the disturbance of the general vitality and of the special organs. Some examples may explain what is meant by this and at the same time may illustrate the close similarity between the experimental and the actual, spontaneous derangement of the psychosomatic personality.

When a person for a long time is subject to dammed up grief and anxiety, a condition may ensue, characterized by depression with irritability, brooding, listlessness, hopelessness, possibly an addiction to alcohol or even suicidal tendencies; gradually the state may progress towards lack of appetite, chronic indigestion,[3] bilious disorders, etc.; there may be headache, a rise of blood pressure,[4] and a disturbance of the heart function.[5] Such a state is duplicated to the most minute detail by a healthy individual who, over some length of time, repeatedly ingests attenuations, prepared according to Hahnemann's method of potentization, of metallic gold. For no apparent reason he starts brooding and becomes depressed, irritable, anxious, and melancholic; he may experience suicidal tendencies or develop a craving for alcohol. He suffers from intense headaches, his blood pressure becomes elevated, and he develops symptoms of heart, digestive, and liver disorders. As soon as he stops taking the gold, these symptoms disappear, leaving him as healthy as before. However, in those provers who persisted in taking the drug beyond the onset of functional symptoms, actual organic changes, often of an irreversible nature, have been observed.

When, however, a patient who spontaneously, namely *not as the result of a proving,* suffers from the "gold-like" disease of melancholia, hypertension, and cardiac derangement, etc., takes infrequent or only single doses of potentized gold, instead of the continuous repetition of the proving, an improvement or removal of his mental as well as physical suffering is initiated. We may mention further examples: Lachesis, the venom of the bushmaster snake, depending upon dosage and repetition, produces in the prover and corrects in the patient a condition characterized by jealousy, hatefulness, depression, deliriousness, vasomotor, inflammatory, and even septic states. Calcarea Ostrearum (Carbonate of Calcium, derived from the middle lining of the oyster shell), though chemically a normal constituent of the organism, when taken in a proving in potentized form, slows the mental functions, makes the provers dull, introverted and phlegmatic, yet at the same time oversensitive, apprehensive, fearful, and anxious, and renders them subject to catarrhal, allergic, and inflammatory states. Salt (Natrium Chloride), in potency, produces and corrects states of introversion, anthropophobia, tearful depression, as well as increased oxidation, disturbed nutrition of tissues, and altered electrolyte balance with water retention, hyperthyroidism and emaciation.

These few examples may suffice to show that the homeopathic literature provides us with a vast amount of experimental data and clinical observations which tend to suggest that every substance represents a force complex that produces the exact duplication of certain spontaneous psychic as well as somatic events. Moreover, in every instance of experimental as well as of spontaneous pathology, we deal with a characteristic complex of combined mental or emotional and organic physical symptoms. This complex is absolutely constant and specific for each different drug and, since each drug can be functionally matched to a certain state of a "similar" spontaneous disorder, it is equally specific for each instance of spontaneous pathology. The only variations within the set pattern lie in the intensity, prevalence or completeness of the various groups of symptoms as presented by the individual prover or patient. Thus, one case of the "gold-like" disorder might, for instance, present itself as dominated by hypertension with cardiac disorder while the melancholia, though present, remains relatively in the background and is brought out only by a careful study of the patient. Another "gold" case, in turn, may be an extremely depressive type of patient, at the verge of suicide, while the digestive, circulatory, and cardiac symptoms are rather incomplete or may be elicited upon detailed questioning and examinations, only.

At this point, it may not be out of place to emphasize that it is not intended to enter the controversial issue of the homeopathic versus the customary method of treatment. The justification for the use of the homeopathic material in this essay is found exclusively in its peculiar experimental arrangement and, consequently, its almost specific usefulness for the purpose of psychosomatic investigation. Admittedly, to anyone confronted for the first time with this material, it may sound fantastic or even incredible. Yet, since it is the result of repeated controlled experiments, it could be rejected only upon the evidence of similar experiments, under the same rigid conditions, which would fail to produce those results. To the best of the writer's knowledge, any such *experimental* refutation has never taken place. Since, on the other hand, he is aware of experimental confirmations from non-homeopathic sources (Schulz, Bier)[6] and also was himself able repeatedly to confirm the experimental evidence, the admissibility of this material appears justified to him.

What could be predicated concerning the functional relationship of the mental and the physical symptoms as produced in these experiments?

The qualitative specificity and individual character of the mental symptoms, giving what almost amounts to a personality aspect to so many drugs, seems to speak against the assumption that those mental symptoms are merely the result of a primary disturbance of the physical functioning. Moreover, the mental symptoms not infrequently are expressed in an inverse ratio of prominence as compared to the physical symptoms and often precede them in time and order of pathological development. Therefore it appears more correct to state that a uniform biologic stimulus (the individual drug) produces a specific response, simultaneously, on the psychoemotional as well as on the biological level.

Gold, for instance, causes weakness, listlessness, melancholic depression and sadness. The prover of Opium also develops weakness and listlessness; but he is in a state of euphoria rather than of melancholia. If merely the generally depressive action upon the nervous system, which is common to gold and opium, were to account for the mental effect, there would not be this essential difference. Similarly, both Aconite and Belladonna are irritants upon circulation and temperature regulation. Both produce acute states of generalized congestion. Yet, whereas the typical mental state of Aconite is one of marked fearfulness, Belladonna is characterized by raging irritability with an absolute absence of fear. Ignatia and Staphisagria both have a general constrictive tendency. However, the Ignatia prover turns into a tearful, moody, hysterical person, whereas the prover of Staphisagria becomes particularly touchy about what others think or say of him; he develops an oversensitive pride and is concerned about his dignity and reputation.

Such fine differentiation and peculiarities could hardly be fitted into the hypothesis of a generally depressive or irritative effect, arising solely from disturbed organ functioning. Moreover, symptoms as strange and, at the same time, as uniquely linked to the "picture" of a definite drug complex as the jealousy of Lachesis, the malicious wickedness of the prover of Anacardium Orientale, or the sentimentality of Antimony, would hardly be assured to be *caused* by the disturbance of some organ.

Not infrequently, mental symptoms seem to be emphasized in an inverse ratio to the actual organic disorder. In cases of poisonings or in provings carried out with rather substantial doses, the mental symptoms are not well defined. In these instances, where the deranged organic functioning actually dominates the picture in an etiologic way, the mental symptoms show nothing characteristic beyond a general depression, irritation or anxiety. When, however, the provings are carried out with the finer dosage of the higher potencies, thus avoiding any gross interference with organic functioning but rather, in a gradual way, affecting the total constitution, the more characteristic and specific mental symptoms begin to unfold. Sometimes, in this type of proving, mental symptoms may even appear before the first physical manifestations are discerned; sometimes their intensity is in an inverse proportion to the physical symptoms.

Furthermore, often mental symptoms appear first and are followed by conditions which we clinically associate with the *results* of such mental states. Aconite, for example, produces a state of anxiety and fright which often dominates the picture long before the appearance of organic symptoms. Later, nervous, circulatory and digestive derangements (tachycardia palpitations, faintness, restlessness, vomiting, diarrhea, etc.) may develop, such as we generally associate with the effects of fright or shock. According to the simile principle, Aconite has clinically been found to be indicated for the ill effects of shock and fright but also, conversely, for acute congestion or circulatory disorders, attended or followed by marked fear. Thus, what we might call, in our example, the "Aconite disorder", namely the functional complex, established by frequent doses (in a proving), or corrected by infrequent doses (in spontaneous illness) of Aconite, presents itself as a psychophysical complex which can be set into motion from either direction, the physical or the mental one, or from both sides simultaneously. It comprises circulatory disorders, etc., resulting in fear; and also fear followed by circulatory disorder, as well as circulatory disorder and fear, simultaneously.

On the basis of these observations, we cannot well consider the mental symptoms, from the viewpoint of the one-sided causation, as merely the effect of organic disarrangement (except for the cases of massive poisoning as outlined above). Rather we must assume a primarily bipolar effect of the drug upon the two different levels of expression, the mental and the physical one:

A uniform biologic stimulus (the individual drug) is capable of producing a specific response, simultaneously, upon the psychoemotional as well as on the biological level.

These two levels of expression appear to be in a relation of what we may call associated coexistence or synchronicity, rather than of one-sided, fixed causation. (Jung, who introduced the term, speaks of synchronicity in connection with parallel phenomena which "simply cannot be related to each other in a causal way but must be in a different genetic relation.")[7]

Yet, since, on the other hand our experiments also showed a definite, close mutual influence of one level upon the other, we cannot yet be satisfied with this one-sidedly dualistic explanation.

For a better evaluation of this phenomenon we might compare it with a relatively simple analogous one, the discharge of atmospheric electricity which produces lightning and thunder. Although lightning and thunder are experienced as differing isolated phenomena of light and sound, their difference lies only in the form of manifestation of an identical process (electric discharge) which they bring to our experience. We usually do not perceive lightning and thunder as simultaneous and often may even observe only the one to the exclusion of the other. However, since we understand the processual, qualitative correlation of lightning and thunder we do not question the basic identity of their underlying force process. Similarly, in our experimental proving we perceive *two* different manifestations (psychic and physical symptoms) resulting from *one* stimulus (drug); in analogy to lightning and thunder they may be observed simultaneously or in a timely sequence. At times one type of expression may be so feeble as to escape notice so that we observe only the physical or only the mental phenomenon on superficial examination. But never is the characteristic qualitative pattern changed which is typical of the given drug.

Thus we are justified in the conclusion that the two responses, the organic and the physical, to the one specific stimulus, must be functionally identical, though in the mode of their manifestation they certainly do differ.

Clinical experience seems to bear out our assumption. We know that mental and physical symptoms are largely interchangeable. Emotional suppression leads to physical disorder; physical suppression (e.g. menses, lochia, etc.) may produce hysterical and even psychotic states. In psychiatry even the term "conversion" state is used to denote somatic manifestations of mental or emotional disturbances. Reich[8] has shown that the dissolution of certain muscular inhibitions and tensions often leads to the spontaneous dissolution of characterological inhibitions. This characterological shift is attended by vegetative symptoms like trembling and jerking of muscles, itching, gooseflesh, sensations of hot and cold, etc. Reich concludes that "all these somatic symptoms are not the result, nor the causes or the accompaniment of the psychic processes" but that "they are these processes themselves in the somatic sphere". Upon careful observation every mental disorder reveals definite characteristic organic symptoms, even as every patient with an organic illness has his characteristic mental symptoms.

Thus the actual instances of clinical disorders fit into the concept of the fundamental identity of the processes which present themselves in a dual manifestation in the psychic and somatic spheres.

So far, our hypothesis has rested on the experiment which was based upon the introduction of a third factor, the drug. The proving experiments have shown that under proper experimental conditions any and every existing substance of mineral, plant or animal origin is able to call forth a qualitatively specific biologic response in a human prover. From the drug originates the stimulus that calls forth the ambivalent response which is always qualitatively specific for each substance. Consequently this "medicinal" substance itself, though it is a part of the nonhuman realm, must obviously partake of the force pattern, namely, the specific psychophysical disturbance, which it sets into motion. On the other hand, the actual instances of emotional or physical disorders differ from our experiment in not ensuing, as a rule, from a drug stimulus. Yet, even spontaneous illness is linked to a specific exogenous drug pattern, inasmuch as for every case of illness a drug pattern can be found the experimental proving symptoms of which are a photographically exact replica of the patient's state, thus suggesting, again, the functional identity of the biologic mechanisms which underlie the disturbances.

The pathogenetic symptoms of the various medicinal substances thus offer the most precise method of describing or summarizing, rather than defining, the dualistic (soul-body) manifestations of the uniform functional entity. The human dual psychosomatic unit appears in a synthetic replica upon a third level of manifestation: the nonhuman substances and their force patterns.

An analogous situation presents itself in analytical psychology. In the activity of the psyche, inner events are summarized and symbolized in the form and appearance of outside objects or functions. Many of these symbols are of a strictly subjective character, and depend upon the individual patient's variable associative patterns. Other symbols, however, are of an almost objective and invariable nature. They have retained an immutable identity of meaning throughout recorded history regardless of person, sex, language, race, nation, or epoch and individual understanding. They appear not generated by the individual person but to be objective, *a priori,* existing entities, independent of the individual's understanding. We might feel almost that they, at times, impress themselves upon a person who, usually, is absolutely unaware of their meaning. For this reason Jung calls them collective symbols.

In the process of symbol formation the psyche carries out a process of identification which links objects and functions of the outer world to the inner soul process upon the basis of what we may call *appearance.* For instance: the sea is the symbol of the collective unconscious "because it hides unsuspected depth under a reflecting surface".[9] Green is the symbol of growing, because growth, as found in its purest form in the plant, is invariably characteritzed by the color green. Birds are thoughts and flights of mind, etc. Appearance, namely the morphological and behavioristic manifestations of living or lifeless objects, thus plays the same role of linking the inner process to the outer as do the biochemical and physiologic properties of a drug which, as we have seen, link the outside substance to biologic happenings.

What reality, if any at all, stands behind this linking of inner and outer process upon the basis of like appearance? The fact of the regularity and basic invariability of the associated patterns, regardless of epoch or individual, suggests that an objective factor must be common to the soul event as well as to the nature process or object which furnishes the symbol picture. At first, we might be tempted to assume that green, for instance, appears as the symbol of growth, simply because it is the color of plants and our mental process associates

31

it with growth on the basis of mere superficial resemblance. Yet, not only do *we* associate green with growth but it actually is the color associated *by nature* with growth, namely in the plant where growth appears in its purest and least impeded form. Whenever green is replaced by a different color it means that growth has come to a standstill, as witnessed in the termination of the plant in the varicolored blossom (seldom green) or in the reverse action of growth, namely wilting. When, in the ascending evolution, the abounding power of growth is restricted by the appearance of a soul life, the green of the plant gives way to the red of the blood, the color of emotion.

Thus our subjective associative processes, far from establishing any arbitrary connections, seem merely to follow what is intuitively grasped as already objectively associated by nature in a creative totality. Even as the symbol is the image and expression, in terms of form and appearance, of specific psychic energies, so is the morphological manifestation or appearance of an object or function in nature the expression and image in the world of sense perception of its intrinsic functional dynamism. The conclusion is obvious that whenever the two energies, the psychic and the outer one, are linked by the identical morphological image, they must somehow be *objectively* associated (namely, functionally identical) although this identity manifests itself in, as it were, a different language, depending upon the particular level of expression, in our example in plant growth, soma or psyche.

In our biologic research we have shown little inclination, until now, to consider an objective connection between appearance or morphology and inner functioning. But in terms of strictest biological reasoning there is no real justification to exclude structure, form, color and characteristic behavior from our acceptance as objective manifestations of an inherent force pattern, and, arbitrarily, to limit this acceptance to biochemical properties alone. Inasmuch as the laws of nature nowhere, permit any arbitrariness, the morphological and behavioristic appearances of a substance, plant or animal *must* represent expressions just as characteristic of the totality of the intrinsic law of their being as do their chemical and pharmacodynamic properties.

An example might illustrate the practical implications of this assumption. Jung describes the dream of a patient in which he sees a vessel filled with a gelatinous mass and points out that, unknown to the patient, an alchemistic symbol is reproduced there. This symbol is the "unum vas" (one or unique vessel): it contains "a living half organic mixture from which an intermediary between perfect and imperfect bodies (the 'lapis'), endowed with spirit and life, will emerge."[10] In this patient's case, his unconscious mind, in order to express the "bringing into life" of a new entity in his soul, associated or identified this state of spiritual pregnancy with what "translated" into physical shape would appear as a vessel filled with a gelatinous mass. That this association is not arbitrary but bears out an objectively set pattern is shown by the fact that the same archetype of form appears, with some variations but identical meaning, in different times, cultures and tradition. It appears as the alchemistic "unum vas," the hermetic vessel,[11] the vessel from which the homunculus is born,[12] the vessel as the symbol of the matrix,[13] the enveloping element within which things originate and receive form, which therefore is identified with the uterus,[13] but also with the head;[14] as the egg symbolizing the prima materia[15][16] which is the aboriginal chaos, or the creative cosmos, as the holy grail[17] conferring eternal life and faith and as the "vas spirituale and honorabile," namely the Virgin Mary.[18]

Our enumeration showed that the conceptual symbolic context of the "vas" principle also includes the head as well as the womb and the egg, since these are the physical organs of birth of spirit and body, respectively. At first, we might look at this identifcation as but an allegorical play. What do we make of the fact, however, that both, head and uterus, are actually morphological replicas of the typical form principle expressed in the "unum vas"? Both, skull and uterus, have the shape of an overturned vessel (our barbarian ancestors even used the skulls of their slain foes as drinking cups). The head contains in its hard shell the soft, gelatinous, structurally little differentiated brain, swimming in the cerebrospinal liquor; the pregnant womb, with its tough, rigid muscular shell, encloses the soft, gradually differentiating gelatinous matter of the fetus, swimming in the amniotic fluid.

The same morphological pattern we find expressed in the structure of a flowerbud, a seed and an egg, as well as in the shape and organization of the oyster: a hard shell encloses a more or less gelatinous, undifferentiated body. Moreover, the provings and clinical effects of *Calcarea ostrearum,* the oyster shell *(Calcium carbonicum),* reveal a dynamic pattern which, in the human organization, specifically affects head and creative-reproductive function and the process of solidification and tightening of the structure from the liquid medium; thus lime furthers and maintains the differentiation of form and structure from the undifferentiated, half liquid medium biologically; and, psychically, it is indispensable for the development of consciousness and mental activity.

We cannot but surmise, now, that a basic archetype of form expression or appearance is represented by the pattern of the undifferentiated matter in the shell; wherever in nature this pattern appears, it is not only "symbolic", but the *objective expression* of a definite entity or functional force principle. In our example, it operates as creating, form giving and differentiating, be it in the evolution of a psychic personality, as a mental process, as the differentiation and solidification of tissues, or the differentiation of plant, animal or human shapes from the primordial chaos of seed and egg. From our understanding of this shell forming principle as the lime forces, we are able to make a scientific prediction: everywhere the processes of differentiation and germination, etc., will be dependent upon a proper functioning of the dynamic forces of lime.

Arriving at a general statement from our specific example, we might say that form expression and appearance are objective manifestations of a definite creative entity. The soul process, when it expresses inner happenings in the visual form of the symbol image, repeats and duplicates the formative process of nature. *The symbol formation is identical with the nature process;* creative nature is the great symbolizer. Soul contents, expressing themselves in the symbols, are identical in their genetic pattern with those physical or biologic processes which are manifest in the same prototype of appearance, namely morphological form pattern. This being the case, a technique similar to the one used by analytical psychology for the unraveling of the symbol context of a patient ought to be applicable to the interpretation of the morphological, biochemical and pharmacological material. The studies of *Natrum mur.,*[19] *Phosphor*[20] and *Sepia*[21] in which this attempt is made seem to bear out this hypothesis.

To the identity of outer substances as medicines, and physical and mental symptoms, we have added the identity of the natural form process in the outer substance as symbol image and of the inner psychic and biologic happening as symbol meaning. We thus have established an *identity throughout of a certain archetypal creative functional force principle* which brings itself into *actual manifestation* in the *most diversified forms,* as the biologic and morphologic characteristics of the various organisms, as the form patterns of the psychic elements and as the pharmacodynamic, chemical, biologic and morphologic characteristics of any substance in nature.

We may attempt, now, to find a general phenomenological law into which these facts can be fitted.

The first to undertake the correlation of analogous, yet diverse, phenomena, using the concept of underlying archetypal entites was Goethe. In contemporary modern science Jung has demonstrated the "archetypal structure" of the unconscious. We shall see that Hahnemann also, a contemporary of Goethe's, instinctively applied the archetypal concept.

Goethe, in order to systematize comparative anatomy, proposed the assumption of an "anatomical typus", namely a basic pattern of an "archetypal animal" (also of an "archetypal plant") "as a general image in which the shapes of all animals would be contained as potentialities and according to which one could describe every animal in a definite

34

order".[22] Those qualities which, upon comparison of the different forms, are found similar or common would fashion the abstract image of the archetypus.

Hahnemann used exactly this method in comparing the symptoms common to most of the provers with those of the most similar diseases; out of those common or similar qualities he fashioned the abstraction of the totality of a drug picture. This drug picture contains every special instance of a proving or similar illness as a potentiality. It is an archetypal image according to Goethe's postulate, since neither any single prover nor any single patient can ever actually exhibit all the characteristic symptoms predicated of a drug totality; every actual case presents but a rudimentary and varied aspect of the ideal conceptual totality.

While Goethe and Hahnemann compared shapes with shapes and symptomatology with symptomatology, respectively, Jung compares soul impulses with pictorial images; their common qualities lead back to the archetypus that expresses itself through symbol and soul impulse. Our study in this essay suggests the possibility of an extension of this method — used independently in morphology, psychology and medicine — towards a synthesis of these hitherto relatively isolated fields.

We might hypothetically consider it a fact of general validity that phenomena which are isomorphic, namely essentially similar but of varied type of manifestation, can be correlated with each other in the most practical fashion by establishing the "archetypal phenomenon" of which they represent the special instances of manifestation.

Whereas the comprehension of the archetype establishes the common connecting idea, the individual variations which account for the manifoldness of natural phenomena can be understood by what Goethe describes as "metamorphosis". As a generalization he states:

> In the fact that that which is of similar concept may appear in its manifestations as like or similar, yet even as totally unlike and dissimilar, in this fact consists the ever changing life of nature...[23]

> We find that the manifoldness of shapes is accounted for by the fact that a preponderance has been granted over the others to this or to that part. For instance, the neck and the extremities are favored at the expense of the body in the giraffe, whereas the opposite happens in the mole. Upon this consideration we at once meet with the law that nothing can be added to one part without having it subtracted from another one and vice versa.[24]

Any intensification of certain qualities of neccesity means the abridgement of others thus leading to a polarity of apparent opposites. Whenever the blossom of a flower is enhanced by cultivation its reproductive ability suffers; conversely, grasses which have the tendency toward particularly abundant propagation have only very diminutive blossoms. Persons who live in a world of ideas may do so at the expense of their sense of practicality, whereas the more practically minded people often care little for abstract thought. On the other hand, an underexpression of one side means a compensatory overstress of another function. Thus the utterly practical and rationalistic business-man may fall victim to unexplainable romantic or erratic whims owing to his unconscious soul compensating for the drabness of his "practical" daily life. Plants of very stubby, short growth often will surprise us by the extensiveness of their roots. Suppression of physical manifestations of a disorder leads to an accentuation of the disturbance on the mental level, whereas the most violent physical sufferings may show but few mental symptoms.

Thus one and the same basic pattern can be varied endlessly by the means of extension and intensification with complementary contraction and diminishment, leading to ever new tensions of polar opposites. The law of complementary balance is the law of metamorphosis.

In his work on the metamorphosis of the plants[25] Goethe demonstrated that the manifoldness of the various plant forms, as well as the different parts within one and the same plant, namely root, stem, leaf, blossom, fruit, seed, etc., represent but variations or metamorphoses of one archetypal plant. Similarly, he demonstrated the various animal and human skeletal forms as variations of one basic form.

Yet, the interplay of complementary or compensatory qualities may also encompass entirely different fields of expression. Goethe draws attention to the fact that, by regulating the composition of the soil, either the longitudinal growth or the flowering can be enhanced in plants;[26] thus growth may metamorphosize into reproduction and vice versa. We have also seen that somatic expressions metamorphosize into physical ones and vice versa. The manifestation of identical impulses upon different media of expression may be assumed to belong, fundamentally, in the same phenomenology of metamorphosis that underlies the comparatively simple morphological phenomena which Goethe described.

Thus, archetype and metamorphosis may appear as basic dynamic principles of manifestation throughout. Our own finding of a common functional force — manifesting itself in the diverse levels of psyche, soma and outer substance — is but a special instance of the broad law of archetypal manifestation through metamorphosis which is the law of creative nature.

The archetypal principle itself, however, is as such inaccessible to our direct sense observation. We can see only its manifestations, e.g., root, stem, leaf, blossom, etc. By means of reasoning abstraction do we proclaim the existence of the common primordial force principle

36

which brings itself to manifestation in those elements. Similarly, we can describe only the manifestations of the spiritual entity that metamorphosizes as soul images, body functions and shapes, as well as animal, plant and mineral forms. The very direct experience of this creative entity itself is not possible to us, as yet. However, exactly the same situation prevails in our understanding of any other force or energy (e.g., gravity, magnetism, etc.). We experience only its effects and deduce by reasoning abstraction its inherent laws of manifestation.

In the investigation of phenomena which we consider isomorphic, it becomes essential, then, to grasp the underlying conceptual entity which more or less perfectly brings itself to appearance in the various forms of manifestation. As Goethe says: "In the deeds of men like those of nature the intentions deserve our foremost consideration."[27]

The method of uncovering these "intentions" lies in the comparison of the circumstantial evidence of analogous phenomena (e.g., extracting the similar elements of drug and disease, symbol and morphology, symbol and psychological problem, etc.).

To avoid mistakes it is essential that only total phenomena be compared with one another. Goethe compared skeletons with skeletons and shapes with shapes, rather than single qualities. Hahnemann compares the totality of proving symptoms to those of the patient and not isolated symptoms (the old doctrine of signatures which represents an instinctive recognition of our basic law becomes a scientific absurdity when applied on the superficial basis of only single attributes, e.g., yellow for bile, etc., instead of total phenomena). On the other hand, a totality is represented not by an endless number of details but by the peculiar, unusual and characteristic general qualities which typify the phenomenon.

By the application of the concept of metamorphosis we resolve the moot question of causation in related phenomena. Neither does the chicken cause the egg, nor the egg the chicken (if we wish to avoid logical absurdity), but chicken and egg are different phases of the metamorphotic manifestation of one organism. Thus the various phenomena of living nature are, all too frequently, linked not by causality but by virtue of their being different phases of manifestation, of a "creative intention" of evolution. Since this evolutionary intention underlies psychic as well as somatic phenomena, we may well look even upon a person's illnesses and constitutional problems as but one aspect of the evolution of his total personality in the same way that we look at his psychological problems.

By applying the concept of a basic archetypus to a practical problem Goethe was able to claim the existence of the intermaxillary bone in man, as a scientific postulate, in spite of apparently obvious evidence to the contrary. Subsequently it was actually discovered. By applying the same law, as the therapeutic law of similars, Hahnemann could indicate the effective remedies for the new disease of cholera, before he himself had ever seen or treated a single case of it. Therefore we may consider this concept of basic archetypal entites not a poetic notion, but an eminently practical approach to a basic, encompassing, natural law which includes, as special instances, the therapeutic law of similars, the psychic evolution by symbolization, the laws underlying morphology and biologic evolution, the law guiding psychosomatic relationships and probably many more phenomena not yet understandable to us.

Progress in science depends upon finding relatively simple basic approaches that can encompass in a living way the fundamental principles which are common to the confusing array of the diverse phenomena, specialities and particulars.

For, as Linné aptly states, "Nature is always similar to itself, though to us, owing to our inevitable defects of observations, it often may appear to dissent from itself."[28]

[1]Gerard Adler: *Studies in Analytical Psychology* (W.W. Norton Co., Inc., New York, 1948), p. 172ff.
[2]Jung, C.G.: *Collected Works* 12 (*Psychology and Alchemy*, New York, 1953), p. 48.
[3]*Ibid.*, p. 169.
[4]*Ibid.*, p. 225
[5]*Ibid.*, pp. 64-5, 169-70.
[6]*Ibid.*, pp. 125-26, 142-43, 170-71, 225ff., 321-25.
[7]*Ibid.*, pp. 84, 147, 255, 413.
[8]*Ibid.*, pp. 193, 225ff.
[9]*Ibid.*, pp. 170, 225.
[10]*Ibid.*, p. 171.
[11]*Ibid.*, pp. 170ff.
[12]C.G. Jung, *Psychologie und Alchemie* (Zuerich, Rascher Verlag, 1944), pp. 103, 247.
[13]*Ibid.*, pp. 187, 212, 249, 324 ff., 455, 459.
[14]*Ibid.*, pp. 278, 325 ff.
[16]*Ibid.*, pp. 248, 325.
[17]*Ibid.*, p. 249.
[18]*Ibid.*, p. 249 ff.

[19]Edward Whitmont: Natrum Muriaticum, *The Homeopathic Recorder,* LXIII:5:118 (Nov. 1947).

[20]Edward Whitmont: Phosphor, *The Homeopathic Recorder,* LXIV:10:258 (April 1949).

[21]Edward Whitmont: The Analysis of a Dynamic Totality, Sepia. To be published in *The Homeopathic Recorder, LXV:9 (March 1950).*

[22]Johann Wolfgang v. Goethe, *Morphologie* (Stuttgart, Collected Works, I.G. Cotta, Ed., 1874), Vol. 14, pp. 173, 206.

[23]*Ibid.,* p. 5.

[24]*Ibid.,* p. 176.

[25]Johann Wolfgang v. Goethe, *Die Metamorphose der Pflanzen,* pp. 9 — 139.

[26]*Ibid.,* p. 15 ff.

[27]Quoted in Rud. Steiner: *Goethes naturwissenschaftliche Shcriften* (Dornach, Philos, Anthroposoph. Verlag, n.d.), p. 101.

[28]Quoted by Goethe in *Morphologie* (Stuttgart, Collected Works, I.G. Cotta, Ed., 1874). Vol. 14, p. 9.

THE LAW OF SIMILARS
IN ANALYTICAL PSYCHOLOGY

In correct prescribing, the symptom totality, as we call it, of the patient must be matched against the symptom totality of the medicine. This totality should not be a multitude of irrelevant details but a certain basic pattern, significant of the total functional unit. Two or three symptoms may already represent a totality, if they are truly characteristic of the outstanding pattern of the drug pathogenesis. This empirical observation points to the fact that in the multitude of observable details certain expressions, notably the mental and general symptoms, are outstandingly representative of the wholeness of a disturbed organism; they subordinate logically, almost automatically, the "particulars", namely symptoms and changes referrable only to certain parts and organs. Attempts have been made since the beginning of Materia Medica study to arrange and classify the multitude of symptoms in accordance with the patterns suggested by these guiding symptoms.

However, we have to admit that our Materia Medica confronts us with a maze of recorded observations which still seem to defy any attempt towards such a logical arrangement. The resulting difficulty is a double one. Practically it renders the study of Materia Medica more difficult by requiring a greater dependence on mere memorizing; theoretically, it leaves us at a loss for a rational explanation for the sometimes rather strange hodgepodge of clinical indications, peculiar general and mental symptoms and modalities in one and the same remedy.

Since the mental symptoms are of determining and over-ruling importance in establishing the pattern of the totality, the conclusion is justified that they must also be a major factor in its formation. As yet, though, we are unable to indicate why certain mental characteristics are associated with certain physical disorders. We are also at a loss to understand why certain substances are related to certain mental characteristics such as Salt to seclusiveness, *Phosphor* to sociability, *Gold* to depression and *Sulfur* to cheerfulness, to mention a few examples.

What avenues can we find leading toward a solution of these problems?

The homeopathic approach is a *phenomenological* one. Hahnemann developed his theory not on the basis of speculation but as the result of pure observation. An analogy was observed between the symptoms caused by a drug upon a prover and the similar symptoms of spontaneous illness. Such an analogy was found to be not mere chance but the expression of a basic functional interrelation between drug pathogenesis and illness.

From this fact the conclusion offers itself that in general an analogy of similar appearance may express a basic relationship since a common factor must be the cause of the similar features, provided that this analogy covers a real totality and is not accepted on the basis of mere superficial resemblance.

The law of similars is the law of the basic relationship of analogous phenomena.

In our attempt at finding a logical correlation between a drug and its mental, general and particular symptoms we are justified, therefore, in looking for analogous phenomena. It is in analytical psychology that a similar phenomenon, that of matching outer phenomena with inner mental happenings, comes to our attention.

Analytical psychology has shown that paramount psychological happenings are summarized and expressed in a picture-language of symbols. Carl G. Jung has drawn attention to the fact that the interpretations which he gives to archetypal symbols have been fairly invariable throughout the recorded history of man, appearing as the expression of identical meanings not only in our individual dreams but also in the various religions, mystery teachings, mythologies and fairytales as well as in alchemistic sources. Thus the interpretation of those symbols appears safely removed from any arbitrary personal preference or prejudice; rather it strikes us as an expression of an actual analogy, or similarity, between the symbol as an object of outer physical nature and the mental content which it represents. A few examples will make this clearer: the color green symbolizes inner growth; red stands for emotion; the number four expresses the principle of wholeness; the sea expresses the collective unconscious; salt the tendencies of the individualizing mind.

What are we really confronted with in a symbol of this kind? A mental impulse or, in our clinical language, a mental symptom, borrows the image of an object or activity of outer nature for its expression. With what right does it do so? Obviously, some objective factor must be common to the mental impulse as well as to the symbol material in order to justify the regular repetition of the pattern. This fact of the regularity of the associated patterns, regardless of epoch or individual, speaks against the possibility that we may deal with associative processes based on merely superficial resemblance. The color green, for instance, may seem to appear as the symbol of growth because green is the color of plants and our mental process therefore commonly associates it with growth. Undoubtedly this is true, yet, on the other hand, not only do *we* associate green with growth but it actually is the color associated *by nature* with growth: namely, in the plant where growth appears in its purest and least impeded form. Whenever green is replaced by a different color it means that growth has come to a standstill, as witnessed in the termination of the plant in the varicolored blossom (seldom green) or in the reverse action of growth, namely wilting. When it is restricted in its abounding power by the appearance of a soul-life, the green of the plant changes to the red of the blood: the color of emotion.

Thus it appears that our subjective, associative processes follow what they intuitively grasp as already objectively associated by nature in a creative totality. Not every symbol association, of course, reveals its objective justification so obviously; our search for its background, on the other hand, may lead us to new insights. Jung himself mentions the fact that the number four appears as the symbol of wholeness and points to what he ironically calls the strange play of nature which gave a chemical valence of four to the carbon atom, the most basic building stone of all organic matter.

Accepting the hypothesis of the objective association between symbol image and symbol meaning we still are unable to account for the fact of our knowledge of the connections expressed in this way. We find ourselves confronted by the phenomenon of an intuitive insight into connections and secrets, hidden as yet from our understanding and buried in the dark cauldron of creative natures and of our own unconscious (since this material is shared more or less alike by all men, Jung terms it the "collective" unconscious).

Returning now with our considerations to the problem of the inter-relationship of symptoms and substances, we note that the connecting threads between outer substances, mental symptoms and physio-chemical organ-functioning lie within the same darkness of our unconscious: nothing but the fact of their objective association is known to us. An *analogy* thus is found between the way a mental impulse is related to a biological happening as affected by an outside drug, and the way the same mental impulse is related to an object, quality or force-process of outer nature, the image of which it borrows for a symbol expression.

In a summary we state:

1. Mental impulses are objectively associated with physical changes and the dynamic energies of drugs.
2. Mental impulses are objectively associated, through symbolical meaning, to outer activities and objects.

The conclusion appears logical and inescapable that the symbol meaning, as emerging from proper psychological interpretation, can serve as a bridge to link and clarify for our understanding the connection of outer substances to mental impulses and to the drug pathogenesis. One would be justified in attempting to use the material furnished by the analytical symbol interpretation as a means to discover the hidden meaning of the multitude of apparently unrelated symptoms.

Some examples again may illustrate this step: We find the ability to produce light an outstanding and characteristic quality of *Phosphorus*.

The symbol interpretation of light as a soul-entity indicates knowledge, wisdom, consciousness, and control of the higher self but identifies these entities with breath and associates them with the physical liver. On the hypothesis that personality control, respiratory functioning and liver function are somehow joined in what our unconscious intuition has grasped as inner light, we investigate the available material dealing not only with the effects of *Phosphor*, but also with the physiology and pathology of light, and we find not only our assumption apparently confirmed by this evidence, but also are able to arrange all the divergent physical and mental manifestations of the drug around a connecting thread in a logical fashion.

Another example: *Natrum muriaticum* is linked to the interpretation of the alchemistic symbol of salt by the symptom: desire to be alone. The alchemistic "sal" expresses the separating quality of the individualized mind and the trend towards emancipation and mental independence. Out of this tendency towards inner individualization the whole of the pathogenesis of *Nat. mur.* can be deduced.

With this new approach we remain true to the homeopathic method of comparing analogous phenomena. Only its scope is extended to include the material furnished by the intuitive understanding of man's collective unconscious, a treasure accumulated over uncounted expanses of time. If this method can stand the test of systematic scrutiny, it may prove of great value to the homeopathic as well as to the psychoanalytical scientist, opening entirely new avenues of understanding for both of them. Body and mind are like two different, yet correlated stages upon which the same directing force, the individuality, enacts the same play in, as it were, two different languages.

In concluding one cannot refrain from pondering over one more fact. The unconscious helps us by expressing inner problems and difficulties, and often the corrective answer also, in the intuitive language of the symbols.

By offering the psychological remedy in a reflection of the inner difficulty by an image from outer nature, an inner disorder is matched with its corresponding similar outer counterpart. On the psychological level the simillimum as a corrective force-principle is presented. A homeopathic approach is found to be the language of creative nature, within as well as outside of us.

We humbly marvel at this manifestation of all-pervading creative oneness.

CONSTITUTION AND DISPOSITION

We frequently speak of constitution and of constitutional remedies. Yet, when we ask ourselves what constitution actually is we find that we are at loss for an answer. A definition like Bauer's[1] "the sum total of an individual's characteristics as they are potentially determined at the moment of fertilization" means really very little because it means too much and is too general. If every characteristic is looked upon as constitutional, we still lack a yardstick to measure what represents the differentiating elements between constitutional and non-constitutional factors.

In my student days we used to act a humorous pantomime called "the hair in the soup." It depicted the reaction of four different people upon finding a hair in the soup. The first one flies into a rage and throws soup and dish at the waiter. The second starts, expresses disgust, shrugs it off, takes hat and coat and walks out whistling a tune; the third breaks into a crying fit because the most awful things always have to happen to him. The fourth looks at the hair, leaves it right there, goes on eating and after finishing the dish orders another portion.

This pantomime, grown out of quite naive observation of the traditional four temperaments, actually casts light upon the most essential aspect of our problem. For it depicts nothing less than four different characteristic reactions to one and the same situation; or to be more exact, three different reactions and one failure to react adequately. Moreover, and this is important, it depicts these reactions in a way which makes it quite obvious that the reactions are preprogrammed and compulsive, not elective. Each individual reacts according to an innate predetermined emotional pattern that makes it impossible for him to respond otherwise. The choleric cannot respond in a phlegmatic fashion nor can the sanguine or phlegmatic person, even if he wanted to, work up a real affect. If any of them tried to do so, let us say by will power and self-discipline, they would, at best, merely partly succeed, and only as far as surface appearance is concerned. But this artificial reaction would be stilted and unconvincing; it would be at the price of a disproportionate expenditure of energy and of a conflict between the energy of the pattern which they try to thwart and the energy of the suppressive disciplinary attempt. For the automatic responses are of the nature of conditioned reflexes and therefore compulsive.

We can observe best if this is true by choosing a more simple example of automatic reflex reaction of compulsive, that is choiceless, character: the coughing reflex. Everybody who has ever experienced the torturing compulsion to cough will remember how, for awhile, one may resist it by a most intense effort of will and energy; yet the more intent we are upon not coughing, the more we must cough. The urge to cough grows, occupies our whole attention; we can hardly concentrate on anything else until at last the repressed impulse breaks through —nay, forces its way through —in an explosive outburst, often of a more violent nature than the original impulse.

While this coughing impulse is a comparatively simple reflex, the temperamental responses quoted above represent patterns of intricate conditioned responses of reflex-like, automatic nature that express themselves regardless of and prior to conscious brain activity, each in their own qualitatively individual fashion.

Such reflex-conditioned reactions of definite form patterns and automatic compulsive nature make up the total of organismic dynamic functioning. They express themselves equally on the level of the body as of the soul — that is, biologically and psychologically.

It is as though the energy currents, the ability of the organism and of the individual to respond to various stimuli were channeled or shaped into various form patterns that for the given species, individual and situation are standardized and automatic.

Just as, upon dropping a coin into a cigarette automat, one gets cigarettes and not chewing gum, regardless of the good or bad intention of the automat (which cannot choose, after all, but can only respond in its own built-in way), so, upon setting a stimulus to the visual mechanism, be it light or a blow on the eye, one gets visual responses, sparks, etc. (Bell's law), since the eye can respond only visually. When one challenges an inherent melancholic response pattern, one can get only a depressive melancholic response. From an allergic conditioning one obtains an allergic response. Each preformed pattern responds in its own inherent fixed fashion.

Thus we may say that constitution is the inherent tendency to respond automatically along qualitatively predetermined individual, characteristic patterns. Constitutional differences are the differences of response patterns to identical situations. Constitutions can be characterized by characterizing these fixed response patterns. Thus we may speak of psoric, allergic constitutions; of *Sulfur* or *Nux vomica* constitutions, etc.

Any attempt to stop the typical constitutional response pattern, or enforce one that is different from the inborn automatism, always meets with fundamental resistances and difficulties; in the long run it proves impossible. The very attempt, more likely than not, will add to the already existing trouble. Whenever the patterned response is one of maladaptation which induces suffering ("pathein") and thus in a "pathological" way threatens the functioning of the total organism, a rapprochement has to be sought, not against, but *within* this individual

45

response pattern itself.

This is a most difficult concept to grasp. But it would be wrong to attempt, as a scientist once said, to "make easy a matter which of its own nature is difficult; then one merely makes it false." This concept implies nothing less than that one's individual life cannot be lived according to any abstract norms or ideals of "normality" or propriety, but only according to what is possible within the limits of a given force pattern, within the limit of an individual's a priori, given limitations, compulsive automatisms, drives and reaction patterns. A choleric character cannot satisfactorily be trained into a phlegmatic response; a *Nitric acid* constitution with its vitriolic violent response pattern cannot be brought into the superficial placid way of living and responding of a *Pulsatilla* constitution. Pathology, suffering, can be overcome only by adapting one's self to one's constitution, by finding a modus vivendi within one's own form pattern. This means accepting one's basic "thusness", accepting that state which cannot be changed. Only by seeking a therapeutic approach on the basis of acceptance of the given form pattern (rather than regardless or contrary to it), can we avoid having this pattern play its worst tricks upon us, and may actually succeed in turning its liabilities into potential assets.

On the psychological level this rapprochement through self-acceptance means to get to know first one's real inborn self. It means to begin to realize one's ingrained habits, automatisms and compulsive drives, the results of very early childhood conditionings or even inborn, inherited form elements. Through their automatic character they are so self-evidently taken for granted that there is no awareness at all of them as characteristic features. To us they are unconscious; to others, alas, frequently all too evident. Realization and acceptance of that part which we cannot change means to abandon many over-optimistic and idealized notions about one's self in favor of a, perhaps at first, humiliating but more realistic acceptance of one's shadow sides. The rapprochement with these shadow sides through conscious confrontation and acceptance can lead to a possible transformation; what formerly worked against us (owing to our unawareness of its trickery, of its demands and limitations) may work in our favor when we accept and adapt to the unavoidable and seek a modus vivendi that, while still safe-guarding our moral integrity, accepts the limitations and demands of the inborn automatic compulsivity. Here the therapeutic act, the therapeutic transformation is brought about through confrontation of conscious judgment with the unconscious form patterns; usually this takes the form of a confrontation of consciousness with symbols which are spontaneously generated by the unconscious, e.g. in dreams. The term symbol is thereby used as meaning the best possible form of expression of an essentially unknown content which, yet, is recognized as existing.[2] The symbol transmits an unknown but highly affectively charged content of emotional impact through an image of analogy and similarity. For instance, in dreaming of a wolf, a message is received by the dreamer that would say to him: "There is something in you like, similar or analogous to a wolf; something greedy or rapacious" (or whatever a wolf may imply to the dreamer). The emotional impact of the symbol has a transforming effect. Confronting the symbolic wolf image brings about a modification within the "inner wolf," namely one's wolf-like character automatism. That means nothing less than the fact that a conscious confrontation with one's constitutional analogon, with one's psychological simile, brings forth a readaptation.

On the somatic neuro-vegetative level the situation is analogous and yet peculiarly different.

Also, here, the therapeutic confrontation is of one's constitution with an analogous or similar pattern. But that confrontation takes place not by a realization of the mind. It is a "realizing," a meeting of the likeness of one's inner form pattern on the mysterious level of biological dynamism; it is a confrontation of one's constitutional state with its analogon in the form of the dynamic force pattern of the potentized "similar" drug. The simillimum is the symbolic representation of the essentially unknown inner constitutional form pattern. By the *Sulphur* or *Pulsatilla* patient we really mean a patient dominated by an essentially unknown force pattern which we cannot describe otherwise than through the *Pulsatilla*- or *Sulphur*-induced symptoms. The drug symptomatology "symbolizes" the essentially unknown force pattern of the constitutional automatism. This "inner" *Sulphur* or *Pulsatilla* pattern, when out of balance (in conflict) with a person's over all total functional personality, whatever that may be, is therapeutically transformed through confrontation with its "outer" analogon. Thus the confrontation of one's automatic intrinsic form pattern "within", with its corresponding likeness "without", as symbol simile or analogon, reveals itself as a universal transforming therapeutic factor both on the level of the soul as well as of the body.

Thereby, we have not explained the law of similars. Like every fact of life and nature, we have simply to accept it as basic, indeed axiomatic, not subject to any further explanation. Any further questions as to "why" are as unanswerable as questions as to the why of gravitation. The absolute and ultimate mystery of being does not reveal itself to the human mind.

We have, however, placed the law of similars into a wider context, namely into the universal dynamism of the transformation of human life through the realization of correspondence; we have placed it into the realm of the strange mystery of the effect of confrontation with the universal simile, whether this is the symbol image reflecting one's

47

true self as a psychic form pattern, or the drug dynamism as a biologic form pattern. In turn, wherever and whenever a will that disregards the patterned intrinsic life stream imposes a repression for the purpose of mere symptom removal, be it in the name of a notion of conventional virtue or of an equally conventional abstraction of average clinical normalcy, the law of contraria is invoked, the basic fact of constitution is disregarded. Repression, discipline and palliation along the lines of contraria have their needful and constructive place. As dominant and exclusive means, however, they are fraught with danger. The way of contraria, of repressive discipline, is a way of life to which the main stream of medieval Western culture has trained our minds in order to teach us discrimination and self-control. It has become an essential element of our rational concept of life in terms of material effects and causality. This one-sided heritage of modern Western man is still so deeply ingrained that the consideration of the irrational principle of interaction by correspondence and similarity is bound to meet with a nearly unsurmountable barrier in the contemporary mind. To a spiritual orientation trained for centuries upon the principle of "tolle causam", the overcoming of suffering through accepting and incorporating that which corresponds to the suffering, which may itself even induce the suffering, the overcoming of evil not through an abstraction of virtue but through "not resisting the evil," the acceptance and confrontation of one's own dark side, the "salvation through the serpent," which Fritsche[3] called "homeopathia divina," is as yet strange, foreign and incomprehensible.

Thus, Homeopathy is still an anachronism, a premature child of a time that is still to come. The resistance to Homoeopathy is deeply rooted, historically, psychologically and spiritually. Homoeopathy is part of an approach into the mystery of existence that as an over-all attitude would be a necessary complementation to our prevalent, basically materialistic and rational orientation.

This step towards a rounding and deepening of our outlook on life and science has but begun in some disciplines. Its general and over-all acceptance still belongs to a future day.

---

[1]Julius Bauer: Constitution and Disease. Grune & Stratton. New York 1945.
[2]C.G. Jung: Psychological Types. Harcourt & Brace. New York 1924.
[3]Herbert Fritsche: Erlösung durch die Schlange. Ernst Klett Verlag. Stuttgart, 1953.

At a recent symposium on the "Theology of Survival"[1] it was generally agreed that the traditional Christian attitudes — rejection of pagan belief in the divinity of nature and the designation of man as the center with all nature subservient to him — have contributed to overpopulation, air and water pollution and other ecological threats. For several centuries traditional theology has tended to create an absolute gulf between man and nature; by emphasizing the value of nature only as it contributes to man's welfare traditional theology has sanctioned exploitation of the environment by science and technology.

That religious values are basic factors in the environmental crisis may seem a surprising thought. Traditional religion as an outward form of worship has come to be meaningless for many people. As symbolic expression of man's transpersonal values and his relation to them, much of traditional religion has lost its power. But the basic convictions and premises upon which a culture is built are not only derived from but identical with religious conviction, so that like Moliere's *bourgeois gentilhomme,* who was surprised to find that all his life "he had spoken prose", modern rationally-minded men may be shocked to realize that his own attitude toward nature and survival are the expression of religious values.

We have secularized our religion by withdrawing from nature and the tangible world a sense of the sacred. Ultimate concern for the transpersonal seems to have gone into abstract ideas of technological control of outer reality. Technology, production of goods and greater physical well-being seem to have become our Gods. We are aware of the dangers of our poisoned environment and of the autonomous, demonic powers of the machine: what seems more threatening, however, is that in seeing nature as 'nothing but' a collection of soulless, mindless things we have become insensitive to the autonomous spirit, the *daimonion* in nature. We have alienated ourselves from a soul quality which could quicken meaning in ourselves. And, like every alienation, this one threatens neurosis or psychosis to collective man as well as to the individual.

Eliade[2] has stated that the transition from a "sacred cosmos" to the "secularization of matter" has led to a "secularization of work" and, may I add, to a secularization of play and pleasure. Work, becoming ever more compulsive and devoid of creative potentiality by serving exclusively 'progress' and greater physical comfort, has no sense of the sacred to give it existential satisfaction. Modern man, racing to save time for the gratification no longer found in his work, then proceeds to 'kill' this time in the same compulsive way he approaches his work. His hunt for hedonistic enjoyments must be 'successful' but is often charged with guilt and seems without joy. In alienating himself from the sacred, man, the master of nature, threatens himself with the loss of his own soul.

Let us look at those traditional ideas of Judeo-Christian theology which we feel have 'polluted' our thinking. The first three commandments present a deity separate from man, one who fashioned man and chose him for an exclusive covenant with Himself. No graven images are to be made of this patriarchal, kinglike leader. He exclusively is to be worshipped. The sacred is severely limited to abstract "spirit", while experiencing the sacred in concrete, material manifestations such as groves, animals or objects of imagination is declared evil. Symbolic imagination is banished.

As the unmanifestable God became identified with absolute good, human nature had to carry the projection of evil — an expression of the implacable enmity between the patriarchal and the pagan matriarchal Great Mother. For *mater,* which is matter, means the feminine, the joyful experience of matter in sensuous ecstasy, the instinctive flesh. As nature became evil and ungodly the realm of the devil had to be subdued and mortified by the godly part of man.

Although we now condemn in Western man this separation from his instinctive side, perhaps we can see psychologically his inevitable need to tear himself loose from the Great Mother. For the sake of an independent sense of personality he had to heed the command of the one and only patriarchal "I am that I am". (Exod. 3:14), forgetting the powers of the encompassing unitary reality, the Gods who are *also animals, plants, stones, places and times.* He had to "subdue the earth" and make it serve the I. These changes of the religious outlook can be understood psychologically as the evolution from a relatively undifferentiated state to a more separate, individuated stand.

Our empirical contemporary ego operates in terms of separateness, rational reflection and the urge to control. Identity of the ego is based upon the feeling of separateness in space and time, subject and object, and even among objects themselves. It perceives interconnections in terms of time sequence, of one separate entity 'causing' another entity to react. Its frame of reference is one of rationality, of a 'why' and 'wherefore' which are directly demonstrable through sense perception. Thus the ego complex tends to operate in terms of 'enlightenment' by directly perceptible cause and effect relations devoid of psychic intangibles, and by will, i.e., aggressive power control. The ego asserts its will against obstacles, difficulties and adversaries which are projected upon the world or even parts of oneself (emotions, instincts, drives). Life is seen as a power struggle in a world of separate entities with a seeming survival of the fittest. And even that survival, through development by mutation of superior qualities, is seen as accidental, rather than organically integrated into the cosmos.

Within the discipline of depth psychology we have learned that when the differentiation between ego and unconscious goes too far—to the point of estrangement—it spells an alienation which may lead to fragmentation of the personality and psychic breakdown. This threat seems paralleled in developments in the world at large. To the earlier instinctual 'all' identity we cannot return; to renounce the level of our consciousness, were it possible, would be to regress to a past primitive stage. We must attempt to understand *the connection between our biopsychological organism and the containing fields which envelop it,* so that a conscious relationship may be developed between them. Toward this end it may be helpful to reconsider those earlier visions of a man-world unitary reality, but which have been repressed by traditional Judeo-Christian thought.

A Unitary Field Encompassing Nature and Man

The non-Christian East and the pre-Christian pagan view the world not in terms of transcendence but of immanence. The Creator is seen not apart from, but as 'powers' of, His creature; or, as we would say, He is its energy configurations. These powers are the motivators or directors *inherent* in the various manifestations of reality, human as well as non-human. Nature and man are the 'visibilities' of the Gods.

Throughout the ages this viewpoint has found its most pragmatic application in alchemy. As Jung has shown, alchemy is a lore of the psyche as well as of nature, and also concerns itself with a practical method of transformation. The "Golden Treatise of Hermes" supposedly speaks of the "body of metals" as "domiciles of their spirits" from which these spirits can be extracted when their terrestial substance is by degrees made thin". Paracelsus, the famous sixteenth-century physician-alchemist, speaks of man as a "microcosmos", an interaction of processes and entities which correspond to and interact with their analogon in the "macrocosmos". Man is:

> . . .heaven and earth, and lower spheres, the four elements and whatever is within them, wherefore he is properly called by the name of microcosmos for he is the whole world. . .Know then that there is also within man in his body a starry firmament with a mighty course of planets and stars that have exaltations, conjunctions and oppositions[3]. . .The heart is the sun; and as the sun acts upon the earth and upon itself so also acts the heart upon the body and upon itself. And though its shine is not that of the sun yet it is the shine of the body, for the body must be satisfied to have the heart as its sun.[4]

Paracelsus carries that correspondence through the other planets and, in principle at least, through all natural substances. Macrocosmic outer and microcosmic inner principles complement and correct each other; they are like yet unlike, polar within a common dynamism:

> Another is the illness and another are the elements. The elements are not ill, the body falls ill. Thus scorpio cures its scorpio [within], realgar [arsenic] its realgar, mercurius its mercurius...heart its heart...[5]

Nearer our time, Goethe, one of the first 'archetypalists' because he was a naturalist in addition to being a poet and statesman, expressed similar ideas in his morphological studies. For he saw the various corresponding phenomena as manifestations of archetypal or *Ur* phenomena in an everchanging play of balance and imbalance. From such examples emerges a world picture that operates in terms of form-dynamics which shape both nature and man through the metamorphoses of grand themes moving in mutual interaction and complementation[6].

Is it possible for scientific thought to encompass such views? Until the Einsteinian revolution of physics the answer would have been definitely negative. Post-Einsteinian science, however, holds a view of a world which operates in terms of energy activity and process, or what one might call the differentiation of spacetime in terms of fields.

> Nature is a theatre for the interrelations of activities. All things change, the activities and their interrelations...In the place of the Aristotelian notion of the procession of forms, it [the new physics] has substituted the notion of the forms of process.[7]

Consequently we now find within the modern scientific world view the realization that

> Any local agitation shakes the whole universe. The distant effects are minute but they are there...In the modern concept the group of agitatives which we term matter is fused into its environment. There is no possibility of a detached, self-contained existence.[8]

And again,

> Since *all* properties of an elementary, material particle...belong to the surrounding field rather than to the substantial nucleus at the field center, the question becomes inevitable whether the existence of such a nucleus is not a presumption that may

be completely disposed with. This question is answered in the affirmative by the field theory of matter.[9]

The idea of material entities pushed around by energy has been replaced by the concepts of form and field. Let us define field as a configuration of energy, an activity potential which becomes manifest through the behavior or arrangements of the particles under its influence, a form-potential that becomes actual in the visibility of material manifestation. Form, or shape, as the a priori organizing potential rather than the shape *of* a material 'thing' becomes the *basic unit of existence.* These forms without content incarnate themselves, move from potentiality into actuality by manifestation through, or rather *as,* matter.

This view amounts to a *psychology of matter.* We find essentially the same concept of form rather than thing as unit of functioning in Jung's mature formulation of the archetype and, in a more fragmentary way, in gestalt psychology. Both archetype and gestalt are conceived as primary form-dynamics. "There are wholes, the behavior of which is not determined by that of their individual elements, but where the part processes are themselves determined by the intrinsic nature of the whole."[10]

Gestalt psychology demonstrated that our perceptions do not occur as isolated fragments which are secondarily assembled by our brain into images or notions of objects, but that they are patterned from the start in terms of whole gestalts. Imaginal or symbolic thinking, i.e., imaging, the experiencing of form patterns or configurational wholes, is thus an inner expression of our oneness with outer reality. The form-dynamics of the psyche interact with its analogon in external reality.

Our psychological experience has shown that every content of the unconscious seeks expression as a conscious experience. Not only human development but also the healing of psychopathology rests upon the adequate actualization of the archetype. Gestalt psychology speaks of "unfinished" situations as elements of psychological pathogenesis. Inasmuch as the archetypal fields — potentials of meaning that strive to reach actualization — shape matter and psyche into patterns of what is to be, they set the directions of change and development. Our freedom requires awareness of and creative relatedness to their dynamics as fields of guidance and evolution. This becomes possible only by approaching phenomena through symbolic imagination.

Jung defines a symbol as "the best possible description of an unknown content which is nevertheless postulated as existent",[11] a symbol "describes in the best possible way the dimly discerned nature of the spirit...does not define or explain, but points beyond itself to a meaning that is darkly divined, yet still beyond our grasp, and cannot be adequately expressed in the familiar words of our language",[12] Symbolic perception is, then, the experiencing of events and images in terms of a significance that transcends their immediate and so-called commonsense meaning. As the field concept has done in the realm of physics, the archetypal gestalt-field concept helps us get past the matter-energy dichotomy which still persists in psychology as a cut between matter and psyche. The symbolic field offers a working hypothesis of cosmic patterns that guide matter, life and psyche like grand musical themes with variations occurring in different figurations, keys, harmonies and instrumentations.

Jung's concept of the archetype *per se* and its visibility as image, pattern of emotion and behaviour corresponds to the fields of pure shapes and their visibility in matter. The archetype goes much further than the gestalt principle, because it includes synchronicity. The organizing scope of the archetype is not limited to psychological experiencing but includes the behaviour of inanimate matter. Synchronicity manifests the same form-determining reality in psychic dynamics as in events of corresponding outer physical reality. Inner and outer configurations are linked by common symbolic meaning. The fall of the coins when the *I Ching* oracle is invoked corresponds to the 'inner' dynamics, which their pattern dramatizes. But this meaning can be derived from neither the external nor the psychological events; rather, it appears as a superordinated third, like 'pure form', to pattern the evolving events.[13]

To grasp adequately the thematic cores of these archetypal gestalt forms one must be sensitive to the symbolic patterns. Such sensitivity expresses itself in the use of imaging, that primary form of perceiving and experiencing which our secondary development of conceptualization represses and makes seem obsolete. We find the purest meaning-charged imaging in myths, fairytales, dreams and fantasy. There it tends to personalize, treating supposedly inanimate things as if they were animated. These personifications, or 'psychifications', of matter must be approached in terms of symbolic perception, for without this symbolic "as if" we could be caught in primitive animism. However, understood as the "best possible descriptions of the dimly discerned nature of the spirit", these images of symbolic fantasy can be heuristic assets; they can be taken as pointers to a consciousness-transcending state which appears as if it were animated, having a life and purpose of its own. As Kekule's vision of the circle of six dancing goblins led him toward the structure of the benzene molecule, so imaginal thinking can lead to symbolic understanding of those universal structures in which our persons and psyches are contained.

Diversified Expressions of the Unitary Field

Paracelsus postulates gestalts or archetypal patterns which underlie human as well as extra-human or 'material' phenomenology, establishing a complementary functional relationship between them: Sun (and incidentally, gold, which is the arcanum, the material manifestation of the Solar principle) corresponds to the heart and its functioning, other substances to other functions. "The Golden Treatise" of Hermes Trismegistos agrees with that concept, suggesting that life and fire lying dormant in "material bodies" can be "excited and made to appear" by thinning and dissolving their radical sources. Man and cosmos are imaged as manifestations of one reality appearing different only in its visible manifestations.

This may seem simply an abstract philosophical idea unless evidence can validate this postulate in practical terms. I believe such evidence exists, particularly in the fields of homeopathy and astrology. These two fields are easily called unscientific or mystical without being put to experimental test. Because they have accepted as facts the kinds of empirical evidence I am about to relate, they continue to be rejected by the still positivistically oriented trends in modern science.

Homeopathy originated from the experiments of Samuel Hahnemann[14], a physician who at the turn of the eighteenth century was dissatisfied with the speculative methods of contemporary medicine and proceeded to "prove", i.e., experimentally test, about a hundred medicines upon himself and his large family. He held that the evaluations of a drug effect should be based only on the reactions of an average human organism. Since his time, the provings have been extended to more than a thousand substances, chemical, plant and animal, and the symptoms carefully recorded and tabulated in their particular details. In these experiments human "provers", people of average health, take repeated doses of a specially prepared form of the substance until symptoms appear; symptoms which can be observed with a certain regularity in the majority of the "provers" are considered to express the characteristic pathogenic effects of this particular drug. When, in turn, the symptom complex of any spontaneous illness is compared with the artificial symptom-complexes produced by drugs there will be found often an extraordinary close resemblance between the disease picture and the picture of the effects of the drug on healthy persons. And the drug whose symptomology represents the clearest resemblance to the symptom-complex of the sick person has been found clinically to be the most successful drug for the treatment of this condition.

Hahnemann stressed that the "similar" condition was a reliable therapeutic guide *only* when seen in terms of a "totality of symptoms". The similar condition must be seen not only in terms of the clinical disturbance, but also in terms of constitutional, psychological and emotional traits of the patient as a whole — in terms of a total image.

Personality traits frequently serve as a keynote for identifying the therapeutic medicine in physical illness. For example, imagine a condition of dammed-up grief and anxiety in an overdisciplined, responsible or repressed person. A condition ensues characterized by varying degrees of depression, irritability, brooding, listlessness, hopelessness, and possibly an addiction to alcohol or even suicidal tendencies. Physical symptoms or organic disorders of this psychosomatic complex may take the form of lack of appetite, chronic indigestion, bilious disorders, etc. There may be headaches, a rise of blood-pressure and a disturbance of the heart function.[15]

Such a state is actually duplicated, often to minute details, in a person who "proves" metallic gold. Regardless of external exciting factors, the gold-proving elicits a proneness to depressive irritation, brooding and pessimistic moods. Eventually the depressive state may extend to a general loss of libido and suicidal moods. A tendency to alcoholism has also been observed. Physically, the gold-proving produces cardiac and circulatory pathology, as well as digestive and biliary disorders. Surprisingly, the overly responsible and overdisciplined personality tends to be more susceptible to the gold states. On one hand they will be more sensitive and ready to respond with typical symptoms to the experimental proving of gold, and on the other, under appropriate strain they are more likely than an easy-going type to develop the gold-like depressive and physical symptoms. When ill they are more responsive to therapeutic gold.

People prone to the effects of a particular substance may be considered to correspond with that particular substance in their own constitutional makeup. The dynamics of the substance 'out there' represent an analogon to the human functioning 'in here', including its mental and emotional propensities. In expressing this empirical fact, homeopathy speaks of "gold", "sulphur", "calcium", "magnesium", "arsenic", "snake venom", "chamomile", and "sepia" (cuttlefish, see below) type persons, each with his typical physical and emotional personality as well as particular pathology propensities.

Let us look at another example: the personality that corresponds to sepia, the ink of the squid or cuttlefish. The *Sepia* condition is essentially one of chronic weakness and exhaustion, lassitude, weakening of the tonicity of abdominal and pelvic supportive structures, a slowing down of venous circulation, a tendency to hemorrhoids and varicose veins, inflammations of the veins, and, foremost, any and every disorder of the sexual function and organs. *Sepia* is most frequently a woman's remedy; its typical pathology is more often found in women than in men. A typical *Sepia* woman is essentially what we may call an animus-ridden person, driving and driven to the point of exhaustion, cut off from and repressing her feminine balance and intuition. She tends to be hysterical, overaggressive and often homosexual. She may appear to be a masculine woman with a narrow pelvis, an overgrowth of body

56

hair, a tendency to beard and moustache and deep voice. Outstanding is the loss of emotional responsiveness, the rejection of the feminine role both emotional and sexual, a tendency to frigidity, and indifference and aversion to family, husband and children. A compulsive need to withdraw and be alone when under emotional strain (despite a fear of solitude) is coupled with a stubborn, belligerent, dogmatic opinionatedness.

Chemically, *Sepia* consists mostly of a substance called melanin, which is also an intermediary product of the adrenal glands, both animal and human. Biologically, the gonads (ovaries and testicles) maintain and intensify the preponderant sex character; the adrenal glands promote the opposite, the concealed and recessive sex character. Symptoms of imbalance in these two systems can be seen in a clinical condition called inter-renalism (corticoadrenal tumors more frequently found in women than in men) which tends to produce feminism in men and masculinism in women. [16]

These fragmentary examples of homeopathic experiments must suffice to illustrate the peculiar correspondence between the dynamics of external substances and distinct patterns of psychosomatic functioning. External substance and soma-psyche operate here as if they were different, yet corresponding and interacting. The therapeutic response is closely dependent upon the specific similarity. In every instance of experimental as well as spontaneous pathology there is a characteristic complex of combined mental-emotional and organic-physical symptoms. The complex is constant and specific for each individual drug.

The specificity of the psychosomatic inter-relationship is extremely important. Each substance carries or commands what seems to be its own peculiar combination of personality traits, emotional and physical propensities: gold, depression, suicidalness, circulatory disorders; *Sepia,* the repression of the overt, usually feminine, sexual dynamics. Thus we may image a substance as if it had an external personality. I have already mentioned how our imaging or creative symbolic fantasy as expression in dreams, myths and fairytales and creative vision tends to personify. In homeopathy this has happened also. Descriptions of drug pictures depict personalities or types, and we have hitherto treated such personifications as projections upon matter. Yet we may see that these projections actually correspond to a functional 'out there'. In this way they have holistic value, as we may see in a further exploration of the sepia personality-drug picture.

The cuttlefish or squid *(Sepia off.)* belongs to the family of mollusk, all of which represent variations of a particular basic form, namely, a soft gelatinous, unsegmented body encased in a calcareous horny shell. The metamorphosis of this form culminates in the polar opposition of oyster and cuttlefish, with the snail holding an intermediary position.

57

Of the whole family the oyster has the most undifferentiated body. It is completely encased in its shell and is absolutely immobile, since it is attached to rocks and stones. The only visible life expression is the slight opening and closing of the shell. The snail, a bit more differentiated, has a semblance of limbs which it can pull in and out, and is capable of locomotion. The cuttlefish, however, seems to emancipate itself from the passive immobility of the oyster. Its life activity centers in the relatively overdeveloped limbs which cannot even be withdrawn into the shell. A pair of fins allow it rapid locomotion, and eight arms and two tentacles are attached directly to the oral opening upon the head. The tentacles are shot out together with lightning speed, acting like a pair of tongs upon prey.

In comparing the different configurations of the shell-encased body (the classic morphological model underlying the mollusks), one may see that this prototype undergoes a process of eversion: the simplest pattern expressed in the oyster expands and reaches its culmination in the cuttlefish. The cuttlefish might appear to be an extraverted oyster; the oyster, an introverted cuttlefish. The dominant tendency of the configuration of sepia strikes us as an overturning of the form-pattern from which it evolved, a rebellion against the enclosed, immobile, soft quietness in which it began.

In dreams and myths we find the archetype of the contained undifferentiated mass. The alchemist's *vas,* the hermetic vessel, the magical cauldron, contain the *prima materia,* or the undifferentiated creative matrix, in the form of a liquid or jellylike substance. We symbolically perceive these images as the source of creativeness which strives for definite expression out of the amorphous. These images presage birth into 'concreteness', mentally or physically. This symbolic complex represents the earthly, the physical and particularly the feminine or Yin principle: the containing and the contained.

The oyster embodies this principle in its purest form, morphologically as well as dynamically, as the receptacle capable of transforming injury into a pearl. *Sepia,* on the other hand, appears in its dynamic extraversion as an embodiment of rebellion against passive, protective and merely receptive femininity. Yet an absolute overthrow of the originating form-pattern cannot be established. As half of the cuttlefish's body must remain in the enclosing shell, despite all attempts to break free, so the temperamental, sexual and emotional tendencies, which a sepia person might wish to disown, cannot be simply cast off. To further this metaphor, the rather odd shape and behaviour of the squid may be seen to correspond with conflict in the *Sepia* person: the conflict between the receptive, contained and even attractive femininity and the unexpected compulsive animus attack. Like a symbolic description of a psychological state, a description of the squid's behaviour reads:

..particularly when irritated and during copulation a dazzling display of colours takes place...During the fecundation period the female swims at the surface at night, emitting quite a bright luminescence. Males rush on her like luminous arrows...When alarmed, a cloud of black ink is injected into the water... Originally it was thought that the ink formed a smoke screen behind which the animal retreated. Recent observations, however, suggest that the jet of ink when shot out does not diffuse rapidly but persists as a definite object in the water and serves as a dummy to engage the attention of the enemy while the cuttlefish changes its colours and darts off in a different direction.[17]

Could there be a better description of the behaviour of the animus woman? Dazzling and attractive as long as she has her way, and when alarmed, retreating behind a camouflage, changing color behind a tangential, pseudo-issue created by the "dark spirit" — the animus — to detract attention.

And what about the symbolic fantasies attached to *gold?* Gold still carries magic for modern man, incorporating the ideas of wealth, security, power and pure essence. Why does *gold* remain the standard of value? For durability, platinum or chrome might do as well; beauty hardly seems a credible basis. Evidently the mythologem of *gold* continues to move and irrationally influence modern man from the unconscious. The Golden Age of mankind is depicted as the age in which, according to Hesiod, mankind was one with and lived in accord with cosmic law. Separation of consciousness and the cosmos did not yet exist.

In alchemy, *gold* is considered to incorporate the essence of the sun, the arcanum of warmth and life in the heart. Not only a life-creating and transforming energy, it is also said to embody, as *(sol niger)* — decay, putrefaction and death.[18] Hence it represents the *prima materia* of manifestation and transformation. *Gold* represents the fiery principle of consciousness, the Christ as the incarnating God, the unknown manifesting as the seemingly known.[19]

Independently of alchemy, the centering symbol of gold-sun in terms of astrological symbolism and life experience also seems to concur. In a horoscope the sun refers to the *principium individuationis,* the central concern of the person's life — his creative impulses, the central assertion of his initiative, and the direction of his will to live (hence also physical health, especially relating to heart and circulation). Psychologically speaking, it points to the direction of the ego-self axis. Compare with this the Aztec ritual of tearing the heart from the living body as an offering to the sun in ritual enactment of the symbolic realization that life could be purified in the war of flowers by being offered to the higher powers.

The homeopathic *gold* picture expresses that disturbance when the life meaning, the heart of existence, the purpose and responsibility of being are undermined. The healthy 'gold-type' appears to be particularly oriented toward living close to central life meaning and self-responsibility.

Unlike the modern homeopaths, the alchemists did not base their pictures upon clinical experiment with the actual effects of a substance on human beings. Their material is more like visionary fantasy (or active imagination) rising from intense preoccupation with the work and meditation upon the substance itself. Yet we can also see how the dynamics of the psyche as expressed in these fantasies correspond closely with the dynamics of the external substance, the body, and even the dynamics of extra-terrestrial events. For the astrological 'fantasies' fit observable facts and interact with human dynamics when taken as images of archetypal field tendencies.

Recent Evidence of Field Correspondences

There are numerous facts which point to the likelihood that these two examples (gold and sepia) of field correspondences are not at all exceptional but exemplify a multiplicity of specific interactions between psyche/soma and animate/inanimate nature, as well as extraterrestrial cosmic dynamics. The southward flight of warblers has been experimentally shown to be based on an inborn sense of navigation rather than on an acquired awareness of the constellations of the autumn sky.[20] Young birds who precede the flight of their parents were raised in lightproof and soundproof boxes. When released they routed their flight according to the pattern of the autumn sky projected in the planetarium; they acted with confusion once the image was extinguished.

Another example is the phenomenon called "the search for what has never been seen", observed in the inborn recognition patterns expressed, for example, in the behaviour of butterflies recognizing their mates whom they have never seen, or the behaviour of ducklings who recognize the artificial model of a hawk, their arch-enemy which they have never actually seen. (Furthermore, they react to the model only when it is moved over their heads forwards, not backwards.) A similar recognition pattern is seen in the Kaisermantel butterfly (as described by Portmann), which lays its eggs in areas where young violet leaves, which the butterfly has never seen, will grow the following spring and serve as food for the young caterpillars.

This kind of knowledge is found in areas other than survival and propagation. We have numerous examples of spontaneous paintings of infants — and even of an ape — which show patterns startlingly akin to electron patterns, galazies, flower and crystal shapes, the forms of sperm and ovum and the DNA shapes. These shapes in matter express

60

patterns which are familiar to us from investigations of the psyche.[21] They point to an intrinsic inter-relation between the form-patterns of spontaneous archetypal expressions in the human psyche and those of inorganic, organic and biological structuring.

Clive Backster, interrogation expert and initiator of the Backster Zone Comparison polygraph procedure, which is the standard technique used at the U.S. Army Polygraph School, employed upon plants the same polygraph which tests emotional stimulation in human subjects. He found to his astonishment that plants register apprehension, fear, pleasure and relief. They respond not only to overt threats to their own well-being but to the feelings and intuitions of other living creatures with whom they are connected, such as a passing dog or a live shrimp about to be dumped in boiling water. They react to distress signals in response to threats concerning any member of the community in which they live, even reacting to signals of dying bloodcells in the drying blood of a cut finger. They also receive signals from many miles distance. More remarkably, the plants registered Mr. Backster's intents, reacting when he talked about them in a lecture. These signals could not be blocked by a Faraday screen, a screen cage of a lead-lined container, suggesting that the signals do not seem to fall within our electrodynamic spectrum but conform to ESP orders. Creatures without nerve or sense organs, such as amoebae and other single cell organisms, fresh fruit and vegetable mold cultures, yeasts, scrapings from a human mouth, blood samples and spermatozoa — all responded in like manner when tested. Mr. Backster's conclusion is that a life signal may connect all creation. His reviewer, whom I quote, adds "Now we know that plants are sentient and that they respond to emotions...delivered from without, the way is open to establish the existence of a life forcefield."[22]

Gauquelin[23] has summarized a number of studies by Japanese, Russian and European investigators relating monthly and daily fluctuations in solar activity to typhoons and other climatic changes, the flocculation index of blood serum, the percentage of lymphocytes in the blood, the incidence of cardiovascular infractions, deaths from tuberculosis, and mining and traffic accidents.

The Italian chemist Piccardi[24] has shown that the speed of certain chemical reactions in an inorganic colloid and the molecular structure of water are affected by daily and long-term variation in solar activity.

Kolisko describes experiments with various metal solutions which were made to rise in filter papers, singly and in combinations. When they stopped rising a characteristic border was formed; combinations of the substances gave different color and form-patterns. These experiments were carried out daily for over twenty-one years. Kolisko was able to establish that in a solution of silver nitrate the influence of the

61

moonphases can be traced: the silver solution rises in the filter paper forming specific patterns which vary according to the phases of the moon. Similarly, other form-patterns varied throughout the seasons of the year; the richest forms emerged in blossoming time, then decreased and disappeared completely between December and February, appearing again in the spring. Surprisingly, specific form-patterns, some of them most brilliant, were obtained for the festival times of the year at the equinoxes and solstices. Kolisko comments that "strange as it may sound, it seems permissible to speak of a mood expressed in matter" as the image-patterns and colours reflect the mood of the seasons.[25]

Dr. Eugene Jonas, a Czechoslovakian gynecologist and psychiatrist, has carried out far-reaching studies of the effects of the sun and moon on fertility and sex determination. Using the hypothesis derived from Indian astrology he tested the following:

1. that conception takes place when the sun and the moon are in the same angular relationship to each other which they had at the time of the mother's birth;

2. that the sex of the child depends on the position of the moon at the time of conception.

   a) if the moon is in one of the six positive fields of the ecliptic, a male child will result

   b) if the moon is in a negative (even-numbered) field, the child will be female.

Jonas' studies yielded an 83-87% accuracy of prediction of sex in four hundred cases. More recent unpublished reports indicate a predictive efficiency of 98%.[26]

Noting the wealth of statistically observed interaction between planetary dynamics and meteorological as well as biological rhythms, Gauquelin worked out statistical analyses of the birth charts of a number of prominent people and found a high correlation between planetary positions and occupational trends. For example, the culmination or rise above the horizon of Mars was prominent in the charts of athletes, military men, business men, scientists and physicians. Saturn's culmination or rise occured in the charts of scientists and physicians. In politicians and writers he found the culmination or rise of the Moon. These findings accord well with the traditional astrological assertions that planets on the angles, i.e., just rising or setting, or at that point, or its opposite of the ecliptic that culminates in the moment of the birth, are of prime significance for evaluating personality. Mars has traditionally been associated with aggression and hostility, initiative, surgical skills, strength, haste and forward urges. Saturn represents the opposite — deliberation, depth, constraint and limitation. The Moon has been associated with collective drives, emotion and masses of people.

Gauquelin shows that psychological tendencies occur in a statistically demonstrable correlation with planetary positionings. What is most relevant to our theme is that the positions, progressions, and transits of the Sun in a horoscope do bear upon what might be called the central life, will and purpose.

Conclusion

From these few fragmentary examples arises a glimpse of what might be called an operational system in which the formal, as well as the behavioural, elements of matter appear to function as special instances of the containing pattern of archetypal life-fields. I therefore suggest that our experience of drastic alienation from the human psyche, and our experience of a soulless, environmentally threatening external world, are in reality one and the same experience of one and the same separation. Human psyche and external world represent polar manifestations of field-activities that encompass both.

Here we have arrived at an extension of the model of the psyche. For in analytical psychology ego consciousness is viewed as a partial phenomenon of an encompassing personality, a Self credited with consciousness and intentionality of its own, even if unconscious from the ego's viewpoint. The relation between conscious ego and unconscious Self is complementary and potentially cooperative. Compensation between them may take psychological form and it may also appear in physically concrete events.

Now the hypothesis is offered that, much as the ego is to the psychic field, the human psycho-physical organism is a partial phenomenon contained in a cosmic or earth 'organism', a 'world soul', with which the human organism interacts in complementation or alienation, depending upon its conscious attitude. Just as the Gods can redress ego hybris in the psyche with neurosis or psychosis, so they can work their ways in the archetypal field patterns of matter to compensate for man's impious attitude towards nature. Human awareness, attitudes and actions may be of great significance in the evolution of the cosmic organism as well as in the shaping of the response of the 'world soul' — whether it constructively cooperates with man or destructively sabotages, inducing world psychosis and destruction.

---

[1] Symposium held at School of Theology, Claremont, California, April 1970, cf. *New York Times*, May 1, 1970, Edward B. Fiske, reporter.
[2] M. Eliade, *The Forge and the Crucible*, London, 1962, p. 176.
[3] Paracelsus, *Opus Paramirum* (ed. Sudhoff), Vol. 1, p. 362.
[4] Aschner ed., Vol. 1, Jena (Fischer), p. 40.
[5] Paracelsus, *Opus Paragranum*, Aschner, Vol. 1, p. 362.

[6]"Every individual form is shaped through circumstances toward circumstances" yet "in even the most unusual form inheres the archetypal image", J.W. Goethe, *Morphologie*, (Cotta ed. Vol 14), Stuttgart, 1874, p. 177

[7]A.N. Whitehead, *Nature and Life* (Cambridge University Press), 1934, p. 36.

[8]A. Eddington, *The Philosophy of Physical Science*, Ann Arbor (University of Michigan Press), 1958, p. 30.

[9]H. Weyl, *Philosophy of Mathematics and Natural Science* (Princeton University Press), 1949, p. 171.

[10]M. Wertheimer, quoted by F. Perls, *Ego, Hunger and Aggression*, New York (Vintage Books), 1969, p. 27.

[11]*CW* 6 *(Psychological Types*, Princeton 1971). p. 474.

[12]*CW* 8 p. 336.

[13]That non-human-functioning also might be directed by meaning in its formative evolution has been suggested as well by T. de Chardin *(The Phenomenon of Man*, N.Y., 1959). And a similar awareness of an evolutionary goal of atoms and cells has been proposed by J. Choron on the basis of the violation of the parity principle in the asymmetry of radioactive emission of atomic nuclei. ("Physics reveals that evolution has a goal", *Main Currents of Modern Thought*, 23, 1, 1966).

[14]C.E. Wheeler and J.D. Kenyon, *An Introduction to the Principles and Practice of Homeopathy*, London, 1948. See too, H.L. Coulter, "Homeopathy revisited", *Scope* (Boston Univ. Med. Cen. Publ.), Sept. — Oct., 1970: "In every country the adoption of homeopathy by a sizable number of practioners has split medical profession into two irreconcilable groups. In the United States the formation of the American Institute of Homeopathy in 1844 was the direct cause of the founding of the American Medical Association two years later. For sixty years the AMA was vehemently hostile to the homeopaths. Regardless of the fact that many of the latter had graduated from Harvard, Dartmouth, Pennsylvania, and other leading medical schools, they were refused admittance to the orthodox medical societies. Professional consultation with a homeopathy was punished by ostracism and expulsion from the regular medical societies..."
"Although the spokesman for orthodox medicine and its organizations were willing to castigate both the homeopathic patients and their physicians they never conducted a controlled and supervised investigation of the merits of this system. The American Institute of Homeopathy in 1912 offered to participate in such an investigation, but its offer was refused by the A.M.A."

[15]E. Weiss, and S. English, *Psychosomatic Medicine*, Philadelphia, 1949, pp. 430, 339, 347 f.

[16]J. Bauer, *Constitutional Disease*, New York, 1945, pp. 86 — 87.

[17]D. Tomtsett, "Sepia", *Publ. Liverpool Marine Biol. Com.*, Mem. Vol. 32, Liverpool (University Press), 1939, pp. 144 — 45.

[18]*CW* 14 *(Mysterium Coniunctionis*, NY 1963), p. 181.

[19]*Ibid.*, pp. 109-12.

[20]E.K. Osterman, "Tendency toward patterning and order in matter", in *Reality of the Psyche* (ed. J. Wheelwright), New York, 1968, p. 40.

[21]ibid.

[22]Cf. F.L. Kunz, "Feeling in Plants", in *Main Currents in Modern Thought*, 25, 5, 1969 (May — June), p. 143.

[23]M. Gauquelin, *The Cosmic Clocks*, N.Y., 1967.

[24]G. Piccardi, *The Chemical Basis of Medical Climatology,* Springfield, 1962.

[25]L. Kolisko, *Spirit in Matter,* Kolisko Archive, Rudge Cottage, Edge Stroud, 1948.

[26]M. Rubin, "Lunar Sex Cycle", *American Astrology,* 1968 (July), p. 365.

Part II
HOMEOPATHIC REMEDIES
AND THEIR ARCHETYPAL FORMS

The concept of causality, namely the linear association of phenomena by cause and effect, has always been an unquestioned logical category; in scientific work, especially, it seems to us the only possible and thinkable one. To satisfy our scientific logic—the causal relationship of events has to be established before we can reasonably assume an understanding of the phenomena in question.

Thus we ask whether physical disorders are caused by mental ones or vice versa. We ask why a potency acts, why a similar drug removes a condition which it can cause; whether prescribing on the basis of symptom similarity removes also the 'cause' of these symptoms, namely the 'illness.' In attempting to find a logical order in the maze of symptoms of our Materia Medica we have to ask such questions as what causes the 'ragged philosopher,' *Mr. Sulphur,* to have eczemas, and why that same *Sulphur* constitution should also be characterized by varicose veins and an aggravation from heat? What causes what, and how so?

At best, these questions prove unanswerable. But, actually, they involve us in more and more illogical paradoxes. The very law of similars itself is such a logical paradox when looked at in terms of causality. That, seemingly, cause and effect could be reversible — such as emotional states causing organic conditions or organic derangements causing mental disorders—seems equally bewildering. More or less despairing of ever finding satisfactory answers, we have embarrassedly stopped asking such questions.

It has never occured to us that the very mode of reasoning which we have come to take for granted may itself be a barrier toward a real understanding of the phenomena of life. Astounding as this may sound, it is precisely the conclusion with which we are confronted by modern scientific insights. Non-causality, as a scientific principle suitable for a better understanding of nature, has been advanced by the exactest of all sciences, physics, and more recently also by analytical psychology.

W. Heisenberg [1] who introduced the so-called 'uncertainty principle' into physics expresses himself as follows:

> In the statement that whenever we know the present exactly in every respect, we can predetermine the future, it is not the conclusion that is wrong but the premise. As a matter of principle, we cannot ever exactly recognize the present.

The basis for this statement lies in the fact that, in atom physics, the very process of observation itself has been found to disturb and thereby change the course of the events which are to be observed. One may determine with approximate exactness either the course or the impulse of an electron but not both; the accuracy of determination of the one diminishes in relation to the gain of exactness of the other. Never having had a firmly exact premise from which to deduce an effect, the laws of energy had to be formulated in a different way by quantum physics.

Thus we may understand Planck's statement that the law of causality has finally failed us in its application to the world of atoms. The arrangements of energy quanta and the phenomenon of radio-activity are defined by modern physics as causeless phenomena, namely, *a priori* basic arrangements. Statements about the electrons cannot be made on a linear cause and effect basis, for instance, by deducing a certain action as effect from a given course and energy charge. Rather, the laws of atom physics are expressed in terms of a generally descriptive statistical probability which lists courses, energy charges and actions as *coordinates* on equal levels instead of subordinating action as an effect to courses and charges as cause. Thus, a totality of a phenomenon, namely, an indeterminable number of electrons, shares on a statistical basis in the known qualities, some having the expected courses, others the energy, others the action, etc. It is undeterminable, however, in what way a given individual electron may express the general statistical law in which it shares.

Each individual case is an unpredictable instance of a totality of a general law of arrangement under which phenomena are related to each other, not as cause and effect, but individually and unpredictably expressing different aspects of that general law.

In a recent essay[2] C.G. Jung, referring to the above facts of physics, states that

> ...since the connection of cause and effect turns out to be only statistically valid, namely only relatively true, the principle of causality is only relatively usable for the explanation of natural phenomena and thereby implicitly presupposes the existence of one or several other factors necessary for explanation. That means that under certain circumstances the connection of events is of a different nature than causal and thereby demands a different principle of explanation.

This different non-causal principle Jung terms 'synchronicity.' He defines it as "the timely coincidence of two or several events which cannot be causally related to each other, but *express an identical or similar meaning.*"[3] He remarks that in the macro-physical world we would but look in vain for non-causal events simply because one cannot even imagine occurrences not causally related. On the other hand, in depth psychology experiences with the phenomenon of syn-chronicity kept accumulating from year to year in the form of the observation of coincidences of inner subjective psychological states with objective outside events, meaningfully related to each other in such a way that their merely 'accidental' association became a statis-tically determinable improbability. These coincidences can generally take the form of the coincidence of an endopsychic condition of the observer with a simultaneous objective outer event that directly corres-ponds to his psychic content (an example of this is the story quoted later on) or with an event that takes place outside of the observer's field of perception (for instance, the burning of Stockholm coinciding with Swedenborg's vision of it) or as the coincidence of a psychic state with a corresponding not-yet-existing future event which can be verified only subsequently. For brevity's sake we have to omit the numerous observed instances which Jung quotes as examples.

Jung comments that these experiments prove that to a certain degree the psyche can cancel out the factors of time and space and that the motions of inanimate bodies can be influenced psychically. Since distance in no way affected these experiments, the idea of a transmission of energy had to be discarded. Moreover, as Jung points out, the concept of causality does not hold, since we cannot imagine how a future event could 'cause' an effect in the present. Thus, one has to assume, at least provisionally, that improbable accidents of a non-causal nature, namely, meaningful coincidences, have entered into the picture.

Jung goes on to state that in the course of his investigations of the collective unconscious he ever and again came up against connections which he could not explain as merely incidental groupings or accumu-lations, since the connections of these 'spontaneous coincidences' expressed a common meaning in such a way that their accidental concurrence would represent statistical improbability. (For Rhine ex-periments the statistical improbability has been figured out from be-tween 1:250,000 up to 1:289,023,876).

In giving characteristic examples from his own vast experience, he warns that nothing would be accomplished by an *ad hoc* explanation, since he could mention a great many such stories which in principle are no more surprising and incredible than the irrefutable Rhine experiments and which would show that every case calls for its own different explanation, a causal explanation, however, being inadequate in each instance.

One example out of the many he gives we shall render in his own words:

My example has to do with a young patient who, in spite of

71

the efforts we both made to overcome the resistance, continued to remain psychologically inaccessible. Her difficulty lay in the fact that she always knew best about everything. Her excellent upbringing had provided her with a weapon ideally suited for this purpose, namely, a sharply polished, Cartesian rationalism with a concept of reality that was 'geometrically' beyond question. After several fruitless attempts to temper her rationalism with a somewhat more human common sense, I had to confine myself to the hope that something of an unexpected and irrational nature would happen to her, something that would succeed in breaking the intellectual retort into which she had sealed herself. I was sitting opposite her one day, in order to listen to her flow of rhetoric, with my back to the window. She had had an impressive dream the night before in which someone had given her a golden scarab (a costly piece of jewelry). While she was still engaged in telling me this dream, I heard something behind me gently tapping on the window. I turned around and saw that it was quite a large flying insect which was beating against the window pane from the outside in the obvious effort to get into the dark room. This seemed to me very strange. I opened the window immediately and caught the insect in the air as it flew in. It was a scarabaeid, cetonia aurata, the common rose bug whose green-gold coloring most nearly resembles that of a golden scarab. I handed the insect to my patient with the words: "Here is your scarab." This experience punctured the hole we had been looking for in the thick armor of her rationalism and broke the ice of her intellectual resistance. The treatment could now be continued with satisfactory results.

In summarizing his concept Jung admits that synchronicity represents a highly abstract, not readily visualizable *(unanschauliche)* entity. He points out that, since the meaningful or intelligent behavior of low forms of life which have no brain and even of lifeless bodies falls within its scope, it forces us to abandon the concept of psyche as associated with the brain. Rather, we seem to deal with a formal or formative factor of meaning, independent of any brain activity, which expresses itself equally through lifeless things, body and psyche. This again is in complete agreement with the conclusion of nuclear physics, as expressed by Schroedinger,[3] that form not substance is to be the fundamental concept underlying the dynamism of matter. We are encountering here the dynamic of what medieval philosophers called cause formalis, ordering power of an inherent form intent or "entelechy." Thus we may come to understand the psychosomatic interplay as but one instance of synchronicity, namely, of the expression of a formative or meaningful element, rather than as a linear mechanical cause and effect interrelation.

Jung goes further to add that the fact of the 'absolute knowledge' that characterizes the synchronicity phenomenon—a knowledge which includes future and space-distant events and which is not transmitted by any sense organ—suggests to us the existence of a *per se* meaning of a transcendental nature that "exists in a psychically but relative space and corresponding time, namely, in a non-visualizable space-time continuum."

His conclusion is that, in view of the mutually closely supporting findings of atom physics and psychology, it becomes necessary to add to our basic categories of scientific thinking causelessness or synchronicity in addition to the categories of space, time and causality. Just as absolute unformed and indestructible energy relates to its perceptible manifestation in space and time, so relates the principle of non-causality, namely, the inconstant indeterminate contingency, expressible only symbolically through analogy, similarity and meaningfulness to the constant determinate relation of cause and effect.

The two approaches along linear causality and synchronicity are not mutually exclusive but rather complementary. The nature of the phenomenon, not arbitrary choice, determines which of the two applies. In the realm of macrophysics and our consciousness of the daily observable happenings, the concept of ordinary causality holds. On the other hand, in the subatomic sphere, in the realm of the unconscious and in the very activities of the life processes, causality ceases to be applicable and has to be replaced by the principle of inconstant, non-causal connection through synchronicity or meaningfulness.

How does this principle of 'meaning' actually and practically enter into the observable life and psychic processes? The spontaneous, discontinuous occurrence of 'bundles' of events analogous to the quanta of microphysics represents a phenomenon, the biological and psychological expressions of which G. R. Heyer compared to the effects of the 'field' of physics.[4]

A field is described as a kind of tension or stress which can exist in empty space in the absence of matter. It reveals itself through the fact that material objects that happen to lie in the space which the field occupies respond to its forces in a characteristic way. This response is determined on the one hand by the type of the field (for instance, the different patterns of iron filings in a unipolar and a bipolar magnetic field), on the other hand by the characteristic responsiveness peculiar to the object (for instance, a magnet needle responds mechanically with deflection, a neon tube with a light phenomenon to the same electric field. A piece of wood will not respond at all). Thus, the field is a kind of a transcendental entity never directly observable which we know only through the peculiar behavior of the objects which it affects and through which it manifests itself.

Similarly, the transcendental 'meaning' underlying the synchronistic occurrences manifests itself to us only through the objects which it affects and which, each in their own and characteristic way, give it expression. Thus, whenever a 'field of meaning' arises in the course of living existence, or, perhaps we might say, when one's course of life passes through a 'field of meaning' this field manifests itself through events on various levels (for instance, psyche, soma), all of them in their own different fashion giving expression to that same formative factor. Borrowing a mathematical terminology, we may say that the synchronistic occurrence of X1 X2 X3, etc., namely, meaningfully associated analogous phenomena in psyche, soma, outside nature, etc., not only postulates the directly unknowable transcendental factor X but also offers us a way to at least approach it indirectly by establishing through a process of imagination the common denominators of X1 X2 X3, etc. Obviously, also, the concept of the 'field of meaning' is itself but an attempt at symbolic representation of something non-visualizable that can never be directly observed. What Schroedinger says of the atom model equally applies to our concepts here:

> The pictures are only a mental help, a tool of thought, an intermediary means...from which to deduce a reasonable expectation about the results of new experiments.... We plan them for the purpose of seeing whether they confirm the expectations—thus whether the expectations were reasonable and thus whether the pictures or models we use were *adequate*. Notice that we prefer to say *adequate,* not *true.* For in order that a description be *capable* of being true, it must be capable of being compared *directly* with actual facts. That is usually not the case with our models.[5]

In the following, a comparatively brief example is given of how the above concepts, hypothetically applied, might enlighten us about the scope of the 'field of meaning,' a partial manifestation of which we are familiar with in the symptomatology of our drug *Sulphur.* In attempting to abstract a 'common denominator' from what we consider but partial manifestations of the 'field of meaning,' that is from the mental, constitutional, psysiological, chemical, etc., known qualities of the drug, in addition to whatever other material we may glean for amplification from other sources, we follow the purely descriptive enumerative method which Hahnemann's genius anticipated and which now has been adopted also by modern physics. The understanding of the broader formative law of the field may enable us to anticipate the nature of events to be expected—on the basis of statistical probability, however, but not specifically for the given case. Similarly, we may, after recognizing a certain drug picture in a patient, anticipate a possible scope of further symptoms that may arise, without being able to predict specifically for the given case which of these possible symptoms he is actually going to have, if any at all.

Moreover, mental and physical symptoms being synchronistically, not causally, related, may substitute for one another and thus one may appear to be able to cancel the other. Thus we get a first glimpse of an understanding how also illness and 'similar' drug energy, as synchronistic entities of the same 'field' sharing a functional likeness, may perhaps substitute for one another and thus functionally cancel each other.

It is not intended, before an audience such as this, to waste many words about the well-known details of the symptomatology of *Sulphur*. In synthesizing these details into a meaningful relation we may describe a constitution which is prone to stagnation: slowed circulation, insufficient oxidation within the cell and delayed elimination; on the other hand, we have also to describe its extreme opposite, turbulent impetuosity: increased circulation, ebullitions, active congestions, inflammations, states of increased, exaggerated oxidations and combustion, tissue breakdown and neurovegetative overstimulation.

Into the first category we may place all the symptoms of toxemia, offensiveness of skin and discharges, lack of vital reaction, suppressed and relapsing states, air hunger, poor appetite with increased thirst, the venous, abdominal and general plethora, obesity, ptosis and degenerative states, as well as the improvement from motion.

Into its opposite belong the classical ebullitions of heat, burning, itching, tissue breakdown, poor nutrition and assimilation, the weak, empty, all-gone feeling, the hyperthyroid, tuberculous, catarrhal, hyperpyretic and inflammatory states, as well as the general and nervous hypersensitivity, the aggravation from heat, the desire for high caloric and spiced foods—to name but a few typical symptoms.

We find that an analogous pattern of polar opposites characterizes also the mentals and the personality type. One group of *Sulphur* patients are rather non-intellectual people, often of the labourer type, heavy, earthy and prosaic; swarthy, rough or obese. They may even be mentally quite dull, slow and disinterested without any introspective tendencies, concerned only with the material and physical facts of everyday life. Psychologically, they could be classified as belonging to the extroverted, sensory type, a type whose main adaptation is by means of perception and orientation through the physical senses of the immediate material facts.

Their opposite is the extreme mental type, the philosopher, scientist or impulsive artist, concerned only with problems of mind and spirit, of art and philosophy, worrying about who made God, bubbling over with new ideas, impatient, nervy and restless, even psychologically itching and burning, driven and driving everybody else, inspiring, enthusiastic, an inventive genius full of initiative, poor in execution, unreliable and unstable. Disorganized and confused, they are utterly oblivious of things physical and material which they also are not too capable of handling properly. They are careless, unkempt and dirty. In short, this is the type of Hering's 'ragged philosopher.' Living in a realm of imagination and always having to reform the world, they also lack real introspective ability and critical evaluation of themselves. Psychologically, they represent an extroverted intuitive type, whose main adaptation is through the ability to 'smell out,' as it were, the invisible possibilities inherent in a situation; they are the polar opposite of the sensation type, blind to all the material things of today, always perceiving hunches and ideas of what might be tomorrow.

Thus far goes our own immediate knowledge of the person who manifests the *Sulphur* 'field.' If we are to fathom its 'meaning,' we need other manifestations on different levels in order to abstract a common denominator. One source of such information offers itself to us in the experience of this same entity as a purely psychological phenomenon as we find it reflected in the alchemistic concepts of *Sulphur.*

Contrary to general popular opinion which considers the alchemists simply as charlatans or, at best, but primitive pioneers of modern chemistry, C. G. Jung has conclusively demonstrated that the alchemists were the psychologists of their day, searching for a synthesis of human knowledge. Their truest practitioners were seeking the 'philosopher's stone,' the mysterious 'lapis' that symbolised the total man. Analytical psychology describes this total man as the 'self' whose phenomenology coincides exactly with the rich and varied symbolism to be found in alchemical literature and in the affiliated pagan, gnostic and Christian writings. In working with their materials, the alchemists' unconscious psyche reacted in calling forth concepts, images and visions which the alchemist projected upon his substance—namely, ascribed it to the substance as its quality. Whereas, to the modern chemist these phantasies are absurd and meaningless, for the analytical psychologist they refer to definite formative elements of the unconscious psyche; since these are to be found not only in the alchemist's phantasies, but also in the average dream material of people of our own time, they are

76

meaningful and practically applicable for the diagnosis, interpretation and treatment of contemporary psychological problems. Thereby, they give evidence of their psychological truth as timeless, transcendental, meaningful entities of the psychic realm.

In passing, it may be mentioned that the analytical psychologist views the alchemistic conceptions only as psychological projections, namely, endopsychic stirrings naively ascribed to a substance; in psychology the question has not been raised at all whether the substance may not have something to do with the images it seems to call forth. For the modern psychologist, limited in his understanding to the usual concepts of chemistry and medicine, knows as yet little about the dynamic tendencies of substances in terms of constitution, personality and psyche just as the average homeopath knows little about depth psychology. However, by bringing together these two fields of experience, a fuller comprehension of the 'field of meaning,' the psychosomatic synchronicity, may be gained.

To the alchemists, *Sulphur* represented the double nature of the soul.[6] *Sulphur* had a double nature[7] *(Sulphur duplex):* one, the white one, *Sulphur crudum* and *vulgare,* corporeal, heavy, earthly and inimical to the sublime 'lapis,' the philosopher's stone; the other red form and spirit, the fiery sublime material of the 'lapis' itself.

The crude or vulgar *Sulphur* was called earthly filth, corporeal, dense, tough, derived from the 'fat of the earth,' ashes of ashes, dregs, scum and refuse of evil smell and weak power, the essence of decay, corrpution and putrefaction and the source of imperfection, causing the blackness of every work. The other nature of *Sulphur,* however, was described as a spiritual principle, the carrier of light and fire, the soul of all natural beings, the 'fermentum' which gives life to the imperfect bodies, the principle of the generative power of the sun, spirit of life, light of nature, creator of a thousand things, heart of all things, creating the mind and the colour of all living things, the principle of desirousness *(concupiscentia)* and aggressiveness.

Moreover, *Sulphur* was allegorized as the 'medicina' as well as the 'medicus,' the physician who receives an incurable wound. This alludes to the ubiquitous myths of the Divine Healer (for instance, Asclepius but also Christ) who always himself suffers the sickness he cures. In the mythologem the god sends the illness, is the illness, is ill (wounded or persecuted), is the medicine, and heals the illness.[8]

In other words, *Sulphur* embodied the principle of universal illness and the potential of its cure...this is not too far from Hahnemann's phrase of 'king of antipsorics.'

We may attempt now to interpret this symbolism in modern psychological terms. Nothing less than the basic polarity and conflict of the soul seems expressed here as it embraces and is torn between spirit and matter. One aspect expresses the force of physical instincts that involves us in the material and sensory sides of existence, the level of our animal nature which, yet, is the matrix, source and maintaining strength of our physical existence and the stage upon which our lesson of life has to be learned. However, when the instinct side becomes one-sidedly preponderant, a stagnation results of one's inner progress, a corruption of one's humanness through purely materialistic, egotistical instinct-gratification. The opposite aspect represents the stimulus of the intuitive breath of the spirit which enlivens and quickens existence in a constant process of seething and generating process never allows life to come to a rest, it endlessly promotes evolution and development and is always in opposition to standstill and the established order of things. Yet, through its one-sided preponderance, one would lose the ground of reality under one's feet and become oblivious to one's earthly limitations. The person who loses contact with his instinct nature is subject to a psychological inflation as we meet it in the conceit of the 'spiritual' person, preaching, teaching and reforming the whole world, completely involved in mental speculations.

In the elements of these psychological pictures we readily can recognize the elements of the two contrasting types of our *Sulphur* personality and constitution: the stagnating, congested, earthy side and the restless, driving, burning, itching, ragged philosopher with all possible blendings and combinations of the individual elements in one particular person.

Beyond these superficial aspects, however, the polarity seems to allude to the mysterious and intricate intertwining of spirit and matter and the paradoxes of existence which we often experience as moral problems. This is touched upon in the symbolism of the identity of illness: medicine and healer, which looms in the background as a transcendent archetypal principle encompassing and transcending good and evil, life and death, earth and spirit, and forces upon us the almost impossible task of being a dweller in two worlds, rendering unto Caesar what is Caesar's and unto God what is God's.

Unconsciously, this may loom as a background problem wherever the conflict situation is brought forth that manifests the 'force field' that homeopaths or alchemists call *Sulphur.*

What is to be gained by considering the above psychological symbolism? It is hoped that this approach which brings together Homeopathy and depth psychology may help us make a few first stumbling steps toward clarifying some of our bewildering problems, such as the relationship of life and personality problems to illness, of illness and symptoms to the similar remedy, etc.

In the synchronistic, causeless, *a priori* arrangement, the 'bundle' of phenomena that we associate with *Sulphur*—outside events, psychic,

78

somatic, biologic and chemical dynamisms—all seem to express, each in its own fashion, a transcendental meaning that, with our human limitation of comprehension, we can but describe as a conflict tension between the above and the below, spirit and instinct, intuition and physical reality, the flame of creative impulsiveness and the inertia of dense matter, the katabolic processes of oxidation, combustion and decomposition and the anabolic life process of quiet synthesis and reconstruction. When, in a predominantly extroverted, object-oriented individual, the tension of the conflict exceeds his ability to integrate it by finding a point of balance within that would satisfy the demands of both sides—whenever this integrative ability fails—then either the forces of egotistic instinct gratification, inertia, stand-still, corruption, putrefaction and stagnation prevail or the opposite ones of flighty intuition, conceit, exaggerated spirituality losing the ground from under its feet with restless, burning overactivity mental and physical. Whether this disturbance expresses itself as physical illness or as a personality trait, an analogous pattern underlies the somatic illness or the psychopathology; the same 'field' brings itself to expression on different levels.

Obviously, the conflict thus described is a general human one and does not apply to some individuals only. Yet this would be no more in contradiction to our assumption than the fact that *Sulphur* is a chemical constituent of *all* living tissue maintaining cellular respiration (cystin-cystein transfer) and yet the clinical *Sulphur* disorder which calls for it as a remedy affects only certain people. Similarly, the 'meaning' that expresses itself through the 'force field' is, in its widest sense, valid for everyone. But only for certain individuals does that 'field' become activated in such a way that phenomena of a manifest disturbance are called forth in soul or body: To the psychologist this peculiar dynamism is well-known. To give an example merely by analogy: we all have fathers and mothers and may or may not have encountered difficulties in our relation to them; yet only for some individuals does the parent-child relationship actually engender manifest pathology by activating a conflict. The 'field' may be ever present. In order to be manifest, it has to become 'constellated,' as the analytical psychologist calls its activation, comparable to the 'causeless' discharge of an energy quantum.

Psychologically interesting is the fact that Hahnemann supposedly called *Sulphur* the 'king of antipsorics,' psora being considered by him the universal illness of mankind. Similarly, Kent equates psora to the sinful state of mankind.[9] Evidently, we meet here with an example of how the preoccupation with the same object-matter called forth the same symbolic representations as a spontaneous creation of the collective unconscious. The alchemists spoke of *Sulphur* as the *prima materia* of the 'king' sol and as the *medicina* and the *medicus* who receives as well as heals the sickness, meaning the divine medicine, the panacea for the universal illness of mankind. In spite of Hahnemann's, as well as Kent's, *conscious* commitment to the principle of individualization which is the backbone of homeotherapeutics we find that out of the *unconscious* arises spontaneously the archetypal symbol of the panacea, the divine medicine which is to heal the universal illness of mankind, namely, the split between the above and below. Yet, the divine medicine is an attribute of the 'Self,' which is the synthesis and totality of existence. This the alchemists already saw in *Sulphur*.

[1]W. Heisenberg, quoted in J. Gebser: *Abendlandische Wandlung*, Verlag Oprecht, Zurich, New York. p. 60.
[2]Jung, C.G. *Collected Works* 8 *(The Structure and Dynamics of the Psyche*, NY 1960), Part VII, "Synchronicity: An Acausal Connecting Principle".
[3]E. Schrodinger: *Science and Humanism*. Cambridge University Press. p. 18.
[4]G.R. Heyer: *Vom Kraftfeld der Seele*. Origo Verlag, Zurich.
[5]Schrodinger: *op. cit.,* p. 22.
[6]John Read: *Prelude to Chemistry*. MacMillan Corp., New York. p. 2.
[7]C.G. Jung: *"De Sulfure"*. Lecture before the Swiss Paracelsus Society held on Dec. 21, 1947. Private printing.
[8]C.A. Meier: *Antike Inkubation und Moderne Psychotherapie*.
[9]J.T. Kent: *Lectures on Homeopathic Philosophy*. Erhart & Karl, Chicago. p. 146.
[10]C.G. Jung: *Modern Man in Search of a Soul*. Harcourt, Brace & Co., New York. pg. 264.
[11]C.G. Jung: Foreword to Victor White: *God and the Unconscious*. Henry Regnery Co., Chicago.

LYCOPODIUM: A PSYCHOSOMATIC STUDY

For more than a hundred years homeopathy has anticipated and applied holistic medicine by prescribing for the totality of mental as well as physical symptoms. Moreover, homeopathy could make the most fundamental contributions to genuine psychosomatics, since allopathic medicine lacks the possibility of true clinical experiment in this field. For the purpose of scientific deduction it is necessary to show that whenever, in an heretofore normally functioning organism, certain mental changes are induced, they are invariably followed by certain physical changes, and *vice versa*. Obviously, experiments with animals are not suited for this. The mental and emotional attitudes of animals simply do not compare with the human level. Nor has allopathy any reliable and safe method to induce at will in an experiment with human beings mental changes that last briefly enough not to cause real damage to the health of the experimenter. Such an ideal experiment is carried out in a homeopathic proving. In this way, homeopathy has amassed a tremendous amount of reliable experimental material which in order to furnish a fundamental basis for a new and revolutionary psychosomatic science requires only assortment. Without such material, psychosomatic medicine is foredoomed never to advance beyond mere speculation and guesswork.

In the following presentation an attempt is made to extract from the maze of known symptoms a grand pattern of lawfully interlinked physical, emotional and mental states which one remedy demonstrates. In itself the material is not new.

The experienced homeopath knows that what is described by arranging these symptoms of a remedy into the picture of one single personality represents but an ideal grand pattern which rarely is to be found with the same clarity in the given case of any one patient. Such a pattern, however, is always dynamically inherent, running like a red thread through every case that responds to the correct prescription of the remedy.

Symptoms directly quoted from the materia medica are printed in capital letters.

The *Lycopodium* personality has been described as: PERSONS OF KEEN INTELLECT WITH WEAK MUSCULAR POWER, DRY TEMPERAMENT WITH DARK COMPLEXION. This may be the keynote description for their understanding. Here we meet a basic functional antagonism between mental and vital functioning. Physically the preponderance of the mental over the vital pole results in DRYNESS: decreased glandular and lymphatic activity and DARK COMPLEXION as this glandular underactivity affects liver and adrenal functioning;

this in turn results in a lowering of the general tonus: WEAK MUS-
CULAR POWER, GENERAL WEAKNESS AND DEBILITY, LACK
OF VITAL HEAT.

Conscious activity of intellect and brain seemingly depresses or
inhibits the purely vegetative and vital functions. It is during sleep,
with its loss of consciousness that the vital forces regenerate our body.
We know also (to mention another example) that mental exertion
interferes with digestion. On the other hand, the vegetative (autonomic-
unconscious) functions of digestion, metabolism and reproduction,
centered in the lower part of the organism and representing the main
life supporting activities, in their turn tend to depress mental and
intellectual functioning. A Latin proverb says, *Plenus venter non
studet libenter* (A full stomach does not care to study). Most certainly,
a good hearty meal makes us sleepy.

A rhythmical pendulum swing of alternating dominance between
these two poles seems essential for intelligent life functioning. Permanent
prevalence of one tends to depress its opposite. People of a robust
muscular or fat digestive type are usually mentally less active than
people of the cerebral type who tend to suffer from digestive and
muscular weakness and are of frail vitality. The *Lycopodium* patient
presents a special instance of the "cerebral" type with its vitality
depressing activity proceeding from the head (brain) downwards towards
the vital and reproductive centers. Thus we find that *Lycopodium* fits
WEAK CHILDREN WITH WELL DEVELOPED HEADS BUT PUNY
SICKLY BODIES; that its symptoms generally are: AGGRAVATED
FROM ABOVE DOWNWARDS; and that it produces and cures a
STATE OF EMACIATION OF THE UPPER PART OF THE BODY
WITH A SEMIDROPSICAL CONDITION IN THE LOWER PARTS.

In general, children start out with a tremendous store of vitality and
regenerative power. Proportionately their intellectual activity is at first
on a lower level. In turn, the old person shows the opposite balance of
keen intellectual and proportionately lower vital strength. The *Lycopodium*-like disbalance of intellect and vital power is apt to affect
more heavily children and older people: THE EXTREMES OF LIFE.
A child with less than its full share of vital energy with which to
counter its abounding intellect will be more hampered in its formative
and growth processes by this imbalance than the adult whose body is
already finished.

Thus, *Lycopodium* is most helpful for INTELLECTUALLY KEEN
CHILDREN WITH HIGH NERVOUS TENSION WHO ARE PHY-
SICALLY WEAK and for children of LYMPHATIC CONSTITUTION
(depressed glandular activity) with a GREAT TENDENCY TO TAKE
COLDS. Conversely, the older person approaches a *Lycopodium*-like
state by virtue of his normal development. The adult in need of

Lycopodium will reveal a condition which in normal development would be reached but with more advanced years. He appears PREMATURELY AGING, with EARLY GRAYING HAIR, has an EARTHY, DARK COMPLEXION, DEEPLY FURROWED FACE and is likely to be THIN, WITHERED, FULL OF GAS.

A great deal of further symptomatology can be understood in terms of the development which a person of this basic type is likely to undergo. The sense of physical weakness during the early, formative years results in a feeling of inferiority and insecurity. Our Materia Medica therefore logically lists: FEELING OF INSECURITY AND LACK OF SELF CONFIDENCE among the mental symptoms of *Lycopodium*. There is always a tendency to compensate for one's weakness by laying greater stress on one's potential strength. The physically weak but intellectually keen individual will lean the more toward his intellectual endeavors the more pronounced his physical inferiority complex. Carried to the extreme, such a vicious circle results in the "bookworm" or brooding introvert. The *Lycopodium* type leaning in this direction, is likely to be engaged in an intellectual occupation (librarian, secretary, etc.) with a maximum of sitting and a minimum of outdoor activity. Such a "sitting" mode of life slows down the general and especially the portal circulation resulting in the well known symptoms of: indigestion due to liver disturbance and reduced intestinal motility (flatulence, eructations, gas colics, constipation, hemorrhoids, etc.). Nature's attempts at compensation are expressed in the modalities BETTER FROM MOTION, CRAVING FOR AND BETTER FROM OPEN AIR, AVERSION TO AND WORSE FROM TIGHT CLOTHING.

Some differentiation will ensue from what one might call a prior quality of the personality. The finer natures will be SHY, TIMID and CAUTIOUS; they withdraw from the crowd and in a quiet way tend to their own work. They may diligently concentrate upon their mental efforts. They are MILD and SUBMISSIVE and often have decidedly philosophical leanings. In their inobtrusive way they may attain the highest goals of spiritual effort. The outer weakness here turns into inner light and strength. Other *Lycopodium* natures having less inner resources at their disposal, simply seclude themselves from the company of others (AVERSION TO COMPANY) and fall into narcissistic selfcenteredness. A neurotic personality ensues: GENERAL APPREHENSION, FEAR OF BREAKING DOWN UNDER STRESS, MELANCHOLIC DEPRESSION, OVERSENSITIVENESS. Egotistic and self centered they are EASILY OFFENDED, INTOLERANT AND QUARRELSOME, UNABLE TO ENDURE OPPOSITION, HAUGHTY and DOMINEERING, OVERBEARING IN THEIR CONDUCT, MISTRUSTFUL, MISERLY, GREEDY, ENVIOUS, MALICIOUS, suffering from the CONSEQUENCES OF ANGER, VEXATION AND MORTI-FICATION which they are expert in finding everywhere.

A peculiar strain of conservatism and slowness runs through all shades of *Lycopodium* personalities. It is the caution of a person who has learned to rely not on physical strength and impulsiveness but upon the slower pace of deliberation and careful scrutiny. (CON-SCIENTIOUS EVEN ABOUT TRIFLES.) Underneath this deceptively slow surface frequently smolders a choleric temper given sudden vehement outbursts, more pronounced of course in the irritable neurasthenic who is devoid of self control.

A person under mental or emotional strain and losing the support of a failing vitality is headed toward exhaustion and prostration. The Materia Medica lists FATIGUE FROM ANY INTELLECTUAL EX-ERTION, INCAPABILITY FOR MENTAL LABOR, WEAKENING OF MEMORY, CONFUSED THOUGHTS, WRONG SPELLING OF WORDS AND SYLLABLES, STUPEFACTION AND DULLNESS, FAILING BRAIN POWER, PHYSICAL AND MENTAL IMPO-TENCY.

What we broadly call "vital strength" has its organic corollary in the function of our glands, particularly liver and the endocrine system. The peculiar DRYNESS and low vitality thus correspond a dysfunction of the above. Disturbance of liver and digestive functions, combined with the characteristic lack of physical exercise are responsible for the meteorism, indigestion and constipation so characteristic of the *Lyco-podium* picture. The resulting accumulating of metabolic toxins is expressed in uric acid diathesis and the well known kidney and urinary symptoms, thus completing the picture of the "NON ELIMINATIVE LITHEMIC." The lowered function of the adrenals probably accounts for the LOSS OF HAIR, BALDNESS, DARK COMPLEXION and the FEELING OF WEAKNESS and EXHAUSTION. Adrenalin has been called the sympathicus hormone. A lowering of the adrenal function is associated with a relative or absolute vagotonia which expresses itself in intestinal spasticity, slow pulse and vascular hypotension. This circulatory inadequacy explains the LACK OF VITAL HEAT with AGGRAVA-TION FROM WARM AIR and A WARM ROOM as fresh cold air stimulates the vascular tonus (BETTER OPEN AIR). During sleep the vagus function prevails, and the blood pressure falls. Hence *Lycopodium* types feel WORSE AFTER SLEEP, since sleep tends to aggravate temporarily the vascular inbalance. The gonads, finally, when "drying up" result in IMPOTENCY and STERILITY.

In more advanced states we have a person devoid of vital resistance, exhausted, dry and withered appearing old regardless of the actual numbers of his years: TENDENCY TO SLOWLY PROGRESSING DISEASES, a state of GENERAL ATONY and MALNUTRITION and a tendency to CANCEROUS GROWTH and CACHEXIA.

Frequently *Lycopodium* is indicated in tuberculous conditions. It would be an interesting task to investigate to what extent a personality type that, as it were, over-reaches himself in his mental efforts is characteristic of the tuberculous makeup. An intuitive grasp of this fact is expressed in the interesting characterization of tuberculous patients in Mann's *Magic Mountain.*

It may be of interest to compare the botanical characteristics of the plant with the picture of the person who needs it as a remedy.

Lycopodium is a moss of dry and thin growth; it prefers dry forests and heath, growing to a length of 3½ feet but always creeping shyly along the ground. The spores which are used for the preparation of the remedy do not moisten as they repel water (hence their use as a drying powder). They are extremely hard but burn with a very bright flash when ignited. The spores germinate only after 6—7 years. The plant itself reaches maturity with the ability for reproduction only after about 12—15 years.

Thus the living dynamics of the herb itself express the tendencies of dryness, slowness, hardness with hidden fiery qualities and a great hesitance in growth and reproduction.

The testimony of remedy proving and clinical experience definitely establishes the connection between a certain personality expression and functional as well as organic pathology. No attempt should be made at this point to raise the question of etiological priority of either mental or physical state. Such a question would be tantamount to raising the old problem of the chicken and the egg.

NATRUM MURIATICUM

"YE ARE THE SALT OF THE EARTH" (Matthew 5:13)

Jung has shown that the language of biblical, mythological and alchemistic tradition, far from expressing mere products of phantasy or superstition, conveys genuine psychological and physiological facts, clothed in the universal language of symbols and images akin to the language of our dreams. This language is common to all races, nations, and historical epochs and admits similar interpretations of its main symbols and thought forms. Jung points out that in this language of a universal mind, our individual dreams share with biblical, mythological and alchemistic tradition in a recollection of soul-experience reaching back into ancientmost times, into the pool of what he terms the "collective unconscious" when man in his evolutionary infancy stood witness to the secrets of the creation and life.[1] [2]

In the symbol-language of alchemy the term "sal," or salt, denotes any solid substance or principle which has emancipated itself from a solution or union with soluble or combustible compounds; although the term applied to all precipitates and ashes, a foremost representative of the spiritual meaning which was given to the term, as a symbol, must be looked for in Natrum muriaticum since it is called salt, simply, as such. On the other hand, biblical and mythological tradition speak of the sea, which is the main source of *Natrum muriaticum* in solution, as the source of all life and creation. Modern research, incidentally, supports this hypothesis.[3] [4] [5]

Psychologically, the symbolism of the sea points to the motherly principle of the great "collective unconscious" whereas the "sal" refers to the activity of the conscious mind. The emergence of the individualized mind and personality emancipates itself from the motherly embrace of the collective unconscious in its quest for consciousness and inner freedom. Why was just our table salt chosen to be the representative of this psychological evolution? Is it possible to find this "emergence of the salt" in what we know about the physiology and dynamic action of *Natrum muriaticum?*

Natrum muriaticum, sodium chloride, or common salt, is more widely distributed in nature than any other substance except water,[6] and even there it is the main mineral constituent of the greatest accumulation of water, the oceans. It is present in all tissues, but particularly the fluids,[7] and is the most important mineral in the blood plasma. It is the chief regulator of osmotic tension; by its power of attracting water it causes, upon retention, generalized or localized edema.[7] Plants contain comparatively little amounts of sodium, its function of liquid regulation apparently is taken over by potasium which acts as the antagonist of sodium. Animal and human organisms, in turn, require sodium chloride in comparatively large amounts.

Animals that live exclusively herbivorously show an outspoken craving for salt and will travel for miles to the saltlick. Thus it becomes evident that an increasingly important biological function must be assigned to natrum chloride as, in the ascending evolution of life, to the purely vegetative consciousless existence of the plant are added the faculties of perception and feeling with the ability to perceive pain through the instrument of a nervous system. At this stage, which one may consider as the first beginning of a soul life, there appears for the first time the phenomenon of active fluid excretion through urine, sweat and tears. Thus active elimination, storage of natrum salts and the faculties of feeling are acquired as a simultaneous step in the development of the psychosomatic unit, suggesting that somehow they must be interlinked. This functional association of Natrum muriaticum is furthermore confirmed by the fact that it is either relatively or absolutely concentrated in the organs of feeling or perception, viz: the vitreous body of the eye,[8] the nerve tissue,[7] the brain,[9] as well as in the organs and fluids of excretion: skin,[9] urine, sweat[10] and tears.

The relationship of the principal kations in the blood serum of all animals, as well as of man, is constant: Ca:K:Na as 5:10:160. This happens to be a close duplication of their respective proportions in sea water which differs only by a greater content of magnesium. Even this difference is explained by the theory of McCallum[5][11][12] who, in view of the fact that the sea precipitations of the Cambrian epoch show a very low magnesium content, points out that the separation of the animal organisms from the surrounding water, prior to their emergence from the sea onto the land, took place at a time in which the sea still had a low magnesium content. Thus it actually appears justified to say that in the blood serum of animal and man something like the aboriginal "water of life" still circulates. The plant with its preponderance of purely vegetative, absolute life has deviated from this balance towards a greater reliance upon potassium. Where ensoulment takes hold, notably at the expense of pure vitality and regenerative power, natrum, its most important representative compound being the chloride, prevails over the other minerals.

May not this be the alchemistic "emergence of the salt" from the sea which thus ushers in the aeon of soul-experience? What then, is the function of the salt in the soul-life and its subsequent effect upon man's body?

The personality who needs Natrum muriaticum as a remedy is described as taciturn, gloomy, joyless and indifferent to pleasure; extremely emotional, suffering under the consequences of grief and disappointment; heavy with hidden grief yet unable to weep, or crying in secrecy. Desirous of sympathy yet averse to and aggravated by consolation, even flying into passion when shown sympathy. Constantly dwelling in unpleasant recollections, never forgetting or forgiving good or bad, bearing hatred to people who have formerly given offense. Averse to company, dull tactless, offending others, absent-minded, discontented, irascible and easily provoked. Ultimately, haunted by fears and forebodings, states of anxiety, despairing and tired of life.

The accompanying physical disorders of this state of mind can be brought under three principal headings: 1 — Reduced assimilation with increased tissue breakdown expressed in the symptoms of aversion to food, emaciation, recurrent fevers, weakness and exhaustion. 2 — Derangement of the blood life: anemic and leucemic states. 3 — Derangement of elimination through kidneys and skin and disturbed liquid balance resulting in dropsy, urticaria, oily skin and all kinds of watery, thin, catarrhal discharges.

The characteristic feature which distinguishes the frame of mind of the *Natrum muriaticum* patient can be recognized as the emotional conflict of the integration of his personality. He always is placed upon his own resources, either deliberately, as he repels every attempt of sympathy and companionship (averse to and worse from consolation, aversion to company) or involuntarily, through the loss of the beloved person on whom he used to rely emotionally. This state of isolation and loneliness is accentuated by the fact that love, sympathy and communion with others are longed for; yet an inner command, as it were, forbids their acceptance (emotional, hysterical, full of tears, craves sympathy, hidden grief, crying in secrecy, etc.) and urges him on to find the source of strength within himself. This separative urge is greater than his emotional longing for connectedness, he is torn by inner strife. Deepest melancholic depression and despair may ensue leading possibly to asocial, neurotic or even psychotic states (anthropophobia, hateful, revengeful, pondering over old insults, anxious, timid, morose, indifferent, unfit for work and human contact, etc.). Not directly tending to self-destruction (though this is accentuated in Natrum sulphuricum) he loathes life sufficiently to wish for its termination; he is tired of the load he has to carry without hope of deliverance from his inner contradiction. The "tragedy of man" seems to be enacted before us as, in search of his Ego, he separates himself from God and world, thereby delivering himself to tears and anguish, yet he knows he must go on.

Inner radiance and joy invariably go hand in hand with a strong vitality. This interdependence is best observed in children who show better health and resistance in a sympathetic, joyful environment than in a gloomy and melancholy one. Similarly, what we call the "happy-go-lucky" type of person usually has a seemingly indestructible vitality.

The centrally-rooted attitude of dejection and pessimism of the *Natrum muriaticum* patient must disintegrate his vitality at its very beginnings. Without the radiance of inner light the body wilts and withers. Physiologically this is expressed in reduced assimilation (anabolism) with underactivity of all glands serving the assimilatory phase (Symptoms: Dryness; anorexia, worse from eating, better from fasting; dyspepsia; constipation, emaciation; hypoinsulinism; hypoadrenalism; hypotension and disturbed blood sugar balance; extremes of weakness and exhaustion). While the dejection is thus reflected in decreased anabolism, its counterpart of repressed, deeply-burning emotion results in increased "burning up" processes of thyroid overactivity with increased oxidation and tissue breakdown (katabolism). Again it is worth remembering that the good-natured, merry, smug personality, not unduly bothered by emotional difficulties, usually belongs to the corpulent, stoutish type, characterized by a prevalence of anabolism over katabolism, whereas the fanatic and emotionally torn personality loses flesh. The plant also, since it does not yet partake in activities of the emotional sphere, maintains functions of anabolism predominantly. The physiological chain of increased katabolism consists of hyperthyroidism, sympathicotonia with disturbed heart innervation, increased basal metabolic rate with accelerated protein breakdown and oxidation resulting in increased heat production, disturbed regulation of body warmth and chronic remittent fevers (desire for, and better from, open air; chilliness, worse from heat). This chain of reactions has been experimentally demonstrated even with crude doses of salt.[14][15]

The ultimate component of the functional unit of katabolism is the apparatus of elimination. The *Natrum muriaticum* disturbance logically affects the whole sphere of elimination, resulting in retention of water and waste products due to disturbed skin activity and urine excretion (dry, oily, overperspiring skin; eczema; psoriasis; herpes; urticaria; edema), as well as what often are vicarious eliminations through the various characteristic thin, watery, catarrhal discharges (coryza, diarrhea, etc., and, a significant correspondence to the mentality, lacrymation.).

It is feasible to assume that the combination of disintegrating vital strength, tissue breakdown, and accumulation of waste products due to retarded elimination, leads to an overburdening of the reticuloendothelial system, with anemia and disturbed white cell activity ensuing (leucocytosis, leucemia, spenomegalia, chronic inflammatory states). The cellular elements of the blood especially must be expected to belong to the sphere of *Natrum muriaticum* as they are not part of the plant organization but appear only as the evolution of life reaches the level of animal and man. Interestingly enough, even a certain trend to individuation seems expressed in these cellular blood elements as their kation values vary for each species of animal, in contradistinction to the plasma which, for all animals and man alike, duplicates the kation relation of the "universal water of life", the sea.[16][17]

Some of the clinical modalities of *Natrum muriaticum* may appear in a new light now. One is the aggravation during the day time as long as the sun is on the horizon and from direct exposure to the sun. It is as though the sun, representing the supreme stimulus of life activity, would impose too much of a demand on an organism given entirely to seclusion, languor and withering. The challenge of every sunrise to master life anew can not be met.

The other interesting modality is aggravation at the seashore. It cannot well be the salt air that aggravates as salt is often craved and ingested in crude form with little appreciable effect. Rather, we may assume the cause to be a fundamental idiosyncrasy against the sea, *per se,* which represents the phylogenetic force-complex from which, physically as well as psychically, this individual in his deepest secret regions labours to free himself.

To master sweat and tears, toil, pain and emotion moulds the human personality. To find the oneness of consciousness and individuality (Latin: meaning the indivisibility) within oneself, it is necessary to cast off the motherly forces supporting us in the sea of unconscious soul-life. The experience of separation and of loneliness has to be passed through as a stage in finding one's self. Whenever the demands of this transition prove greater than the strength of the personality, a state of pathology is likely to arise which has its remedy in *Natrum muriaticum.* The salt, which on our earth is the precipitate from the ancient seas, is the true simillimum to aid in the precipitation and emancipation of man's Ego from the sea of our collective unconscious. The wisdom of the Gospel words becomes manifest which addresses the men who are to be the teachers and spiritual helpers of humanity: "Ye are the salt of the earth."

---

[1]Jung, C.G. *Collected Works* 12 *(Psychology and Alchemy,* NY 1953), pp. 48-49, 178-79, 244.
[2]C.G. Jung: *The Integration of the Personality,* pp. 103, 216. 1939. Farrar und Rinehart.
[3]E.E. Free: in *Forum,* quoted by Ivor Griffith, *Sea-Inside.*
[4]*The Scientific Monthly,* April 1941, p. 294.
[5]McCallum's Theory, quoted in H. Marx: *Der Wasserhaushalt des gesunden und kranken Koerpers,* 1901, p. 125.
[6]Neatby and Stoneham: *Manual of Homeotherapeutics,* 1927, p. 623.

[7]C. Oppenheimer: *Handbuch des Biochemie*, Vol. 1, p. 26, 1924, Fischer Publishing Co.

[8]C. Oppenheimer: *Handbuch des Biochemie*, Vol. 1, p. 27.

[9]Heubner: *Der Mineralbestand des Koerpers*, p. 81.

[10]H. Marx: *Der Wasserhaushalt des gesunden und kranken Koerpers*, 1901, p. 172.

[11]C. Oppenheimer: *Handbuch der Biochemie*, Supplement Vol. 2, p. 38.

[12]R. Hoeber: *Physik. Chemie der Zelle u. Gewebe*, p. 666.

[14]C. Oppenheimer: *Handbuch der Biochemie*, Vol. 8, p. 291.

[15]*Ibid.*, Vol. 8, pp. 295-298.

[16]Heubner: *Der Mineralbestand der Koerpers*, pp. 7, 53.

[17]C. Oppenheimer: *Handbuch des Biochemie*, Vol. 1, p. 28.

THE ANALYSIS OF A DYNAMIC TOTALITY: SEPIA

In order to integrate the diversified material of provings and clinical symptoms into an organic whole, we assume that the diversity of physical, chemical, biologic, morphologic and behavior characteristics of a potential medicine—namely, a substance of mineral, plant or animal origin—represents but different phases of expression of one and the same formative functional entity: we also assume that this same functional archetypus also manifests itself in the mental and somatic symptoms of a proving as well as in the clinical disorders of the patient.

To grasp the essential principle underlying all the different manifestations of the energy field of a substance, the most outstanding characteristics or unusual features are used as starting points. Those key symptoms through which we try to unravel and interpret the context of related pharmacodynamic, mental and physical functions may be symptoms of the patient (e.g., the aversion to company of *Natrum muriaticum*), physiochemical properties of the substance itself (e.g., the luminescence of *Phosphor*), or life expressions of the plant or the animal (e.g., the dryness of *Lycopodium* or the production of the ink cloud in *Sepia*).

In the case of *Sepia,* our attention is drawn to its extraordinary configuration and the contradictory phenomena of light and darkness which the animal produces.

The cuttlefish *(Sepia off.)* belongs to the family of mollusks which is comprised also of clams, oysters, mussels and snails. All mollusks represent variations of a definite basic form pattern, namely a soft, gelatinous, unsegmented body encased in a calcareous, horny shell. The metamorphosis of this form pattern culminates in an extreme polar opposition of oyster and cuttlefish, with the snail holding an intermediary position.

Of the whole family, the oyster has the most undifferentiated body and possesses no limbs whatsoever. The animal is completely encased in its shell and is absolutely immobile, since it is attached to rocks and stones. Its only visible life expression consists in the slight opening and closing of the shell. The snail is more differentiated and has a semblance of limbs which it can pull in and out of the shell. It is also capable of a, however proverbially slow, locomotion. The cuttlefish, in turn, goes to the opposite extreme of emancipating itself from the passive immobility of the oyster. Its life activity centers in the relatively overdeveloped limbs which cannot even be withdrawn into the shell at all. It has a pair of fins which allow it rapid locomotion; eight arms and two tentacles are attached directly to the oral opening upon the head. The tentacles are shot out together with lightning speed, acting like a pair of tongs, when prey is to be caught.

As one compares the different configurations of the shell-encased body, the basic morphological model underlying the mollusks, one can see that this prototype undergoes a process of eversion: from the simplest pattern as expressed in the oyster an expansion takes place which reaches its culmination in the cuttlefish. The dominant tendency of the configuration of Sepia strikes us like an overturning of the form pattern from which it evolved, a rebellion against the shell-enclosed, soft, immobile and impassive quietness.

The formative principle, as expressed in the archetypus of the immobilised shell-enclosed jelly represented by the oyster, we find again in the configuration of the human skull which encloses and protects the jelly-like, morphologically relatively undifferentiated brain suspended and immobilised in the cerebrospinal fluid; and in the pregnant uterus enclosing and protecting with its rigid shell the but gradually differentuating fetal substance. The analogous tendency of function lies in the general ability of walling off and protecting the inside against the outside. Biologically, this means resistance against infection and the tightening of the tissues against the overflow of liquids. When this function fails we have a susceptibility to infection and the exudative diathesis, both of which are typical for the patient who needs *Calcarea carbonica* (potentized oyster shell). Psychologically, introversion and walling oneself off mean separating and individualizing oneself towards the world from without and from within. Even as the conscious function of the brain is dependent upon its being walled off by the hard skull, so in the functional activity of the soul the personal consciousness, the ego, emerges from primordial unconsciousness by the process of walling off and separating.

The pattern of the shell-enclosed softness appears also as the alchemistic *"vas"* or "hermetic vessel" containing the prima materia, the undifferentiated creative matrix, as well as in modern dreams. All these patterns are variations of the same form principle which represents the source of physical or spiritual creativeness from which the central self can strive for its expression out of the amorphous.[1] Therefore the "vas" principle is inherent in the head[2] but also, representing the matrix, in the uterus,[3] the place of physical creation. As a general tendency this form complex also represents the earthly, physical and, particularly, the feminine principle.[4]

This principle in its purest, undisturbed form is embodied in the oyster, as is attested by the pathogenesis of *Calcarea carbonica.* The dynamic life expression of *Sepia,* on the other hand, which turns introversion into extroversion, thus basically rebels against the contemplative, passive, protected femininity.

Yet, an absolutely complete overthrow of the form pattern from which it originates cannot be accomplished. Even as a half of the cuttlefish's body must remain within the enclosing shell, in spite of all attempts to break loose, so also the temperamental, sexual and emotional tendencies which one would disown cannot simply be cast off; they can only be slowly and gradually transformed by developing a conscious understanding with which to complement the world of instinctive feeling which is woman's primary expression and experience. Wherever the gradual expansion gives way to a violent, protesting attitude, repression takes the place of gradual transformation and pathology arises. Challenge to and repression of the quiet, contemplative and receptive feminine qualities, symbolized by the "creative vessel," thus become the keynotes of the *Sepia* pathology.

Repressed qualities continue in existence. They gain, moreover, a negative perverted rule over the manifest functioning. Biologically, the repressed sex function distorts the whole of the life activities of the body. It brings about circulatory and congestive disorders (stasis), as well as a state of general ridigity and spasticity, involving any voluntary and involuntary muscle group and organ, along with a state of nervous hyperirritability.[5] Emotionally, the repression of the sexual and feminine traits, leads to anxiety, restlessness, depressive states, opinionated dogmatism and incontrollable, erratic, unreasonable and contradictory neurasthenic conditions.

Specifically, the "masculine protest," if we may use the psychoanalytic term, makes the woman who repressed her femininity a bustling, nervous, fidgety and opinionated shrew. The man who would repress (or fails to develop) his feminine side becomes hardened, mean, egotistical and narrow-minded; he may fall victim to unaccountable emotional or even hysterical impulses when the dammed up function suddenly takes its revenge. We shall later see how all these well known *Sepia* traits find their corroboration in the disturbance of the ductless glands representing the manifestation of the same process in its biological metamorphosis.

In passing, we may point to the fact that the nonacceptance of one's being is the expression of a highly individualistic attitude. Probably upon this fact rests the complementary relationship between *Sepia* and *Natrum muriaticum,* the latter representing the emancipating force of the individual personality.[6] In differentiating the two, one might feel, however, that the *Natrum muriaticum* personality tends to be asocial in consequence of finding himself emotionally isolated by circumstances and inner needs; *Sepia's* isolation bears much more the mark of either deliberate withdrawal and willful moodiness or of a state of utter vital exhaustion demanding solitude to nurse one's wounds.

The problematical attitude towards the feminine principle, as expressed in the morphological archetype, is complemented by a similar polar tension in biological functioning in respect to light and darkness. The following is a quotation from a description of the cuttlefish:[7]

> "Particularly when irritated and during copulation a dazzling display of colours takes place.... During the fecundation period the female swims at the surface at night, emitting quite a bright luminescence. Males rush on her like luminous arrows.... When alarmed, a cloud of black ink is injected into the water.... Originally it was thought that the ink formed a smoke screen behind which the animal retreated. Recent observations, however, suggest that the jet of ink when shot out does not diffuse rapidly but persists as a definite object in the water and serves as a dummy to engage the attention of the enemy while the cuttlefish changes its colour and darts off in a different direction."

This ink, which in its dried form furnishes our medicine, is essentially melanin[8, 9] and, interestingly enough, has a very high content of sulphur[8] and calcium salts.[9]

Sepia thus has the quality of luminescence. It shares this ability to generate light with the inorganic *Phosphor*. In another essay, the pathogenesis of *Phosphor* in the human organisation is explained as the disturbed metamorphosis of the light principle throughout the soul and body levels.[10] As on the morphological plane *Sepia* evolves the polar antithesis to the creative feminine principle of the oyster, so upon the functional level it incorporates the activity of light, yet also develops its polar counterpart, the dark double. The study of *Phosphor*[10] showed that on the soul level light manifests itself as consciousness, intellect and self control; biologically it expresses itself in general vitality, blood formation and firmness of the physical structure with a particular effect upon the adrenal glands and the portal as well as the respiratory system. This patern is largely shared by *Sepia* which, clinically, is complementary to *Phosphor*.

Darkness, on the other hand, represents the unconscious, feminine, earthly principle.[11] What, however, underlies the force process by which the dark double, the direct antithesis to the light forces inherent in *Sepia*, is projected into the foreground? It is suggested in another essay[12] that we might hypothetically consider biologic and morphologic phenomena as determined by nature's tendency to give objective form in its manifestation to tendencies which we otherwise experience through symbols; thus nature, the great symbolizer, would invite an approach of interpretation analogous to the technique of analytical psychology. If we proceed upon this hypothesis, we may say that under stress the darkness (namely, the unconscious) is projected and occupies the foreground. The individual as we know him "changes colour" and becomes completely removed from our sight.

In a most interesting and fascinating way C. Jung describes this occurrence as an actual psychological situation.[13]

All of a man's traits become visible under the stress of an emotion which affords the ideal condition for the manifestation of unconscious contents. Under its possession one is "beside oneself" and the *unconscious gets a chance to occupy the foreground.** As a matter of fact the emotion *is* the intrusion of an unconscious personality.... To the primitive mind, a man who is seized by a strong emotion is possessed by a devil or a spirit.... The character that summarizes a person's uncontrolled emotional manifestation consists, in the first place, of his inferior qualities or peculiarities. Even people we like and appreciate suffer from certain imperfections of character that have to be taken into the bargain. When people are not at their best such flaws become clearly visible. I have called the inferior or less commendable part of a person the *shadow.**... But the shadow is not all that becomes manifest in emotional disturbance; and it is not sufficient to explain why a man has the rather definite feeling that "he is not himself" or that "he is beside himself." There is at such times a peculiar strangeness about a man, which we positively dislike to attribute to him in our ordinary thought of him....

The strangeness is due to the emergence of a *different character,** one that we hesitate to ascribe to the ego personality....If we compare a number of emotional events, we can easily see that the same character reappears in every one of them. For this reason we can attribute continuity to the unconscious personality and ascribe to it the emotional intrusions....

When people are at their best there is not much chance of seeing anything of their other side. But when you observe a man when he is caught in a mood you find him to be a different person. The observer who has sharpened his eyes and acquired a good deal of practical experience begins to discover symptoms of the man in the woman and the woman in the man. Sometimes the change is quite remarkable; a man who is ordinarily altruistic, generous, amiable and intelligent becomes, when a certain mood seizes him, a slightly mean, nastily egotistical and illogically prejudiced character. A woman of a usually kind and peaceable disposition becomes an argumentative, obstinate, narrowminded shrew. It is easy to observe that women at a more advanced age develop masculine qualities, develop a mustache, acquire a rather acute and sometimes obstinate mind and often develop a deeper voice. Men of advanced age, on the contrary become mellow, "lovely" old men, soft, kind to children, sentimental and rather emotional. Their anatomical forms become rounded, they take interest in family and homelife, in genealogy, gossip and so on. It is by no means rare for the wife to take over business responsibilities in later life while the husband plays merely a helpful role....

Should you study this world wide experience with due attention, and regard the "other side" as a trait of character, you will produce a picture that shows what I mean by the "anima," the *woman in a man,** and the "animus," the *man in a woman.**

It may strike the reader that my description of the shadow does not markedly differ from my picture of the anima. This is due to the fact that I have spoken only of the immediate and superficial aspects of these figures.

It is, however, just this "immediate and superficial aspect" in which "shadow" is still conjoined to the contra-sexual soul impulse with which we deal in the *Sepia* phenomenology. If we use Jung's terminology, the "shadow" denotes man's "alter darker ego," namely, the inferior, unacceptable, undeveloped or suppressed part of his being. It has found its symbolic representations in the figure of Satan, the devil, the "dark double," the spirit or demon of evil, Shakespeare's Caliban, etc.

Such a "dark double" is concretely produced by the "emotional eruption" of the cuttlefish. The anima or animus with which the shadow appears conjoined in this immediate superficial aspect is the heterosexual psychic driving impulse. Jung stresses the fact that the driving and leading personality aspect of everybody's unconscious soul life bears the character marks of the opposite sex; within the unconscious it thus performs a function which is balancing and complementary to the manifest, conscious attitude.

The following quotations from analytical literature[14, 15] may be helpful for a better understanding:

The archetypal figure of the soul image stands for the respective contra-sexual portion of the psyche, showing partly how our

---

*Italics are mine—E.W.

personal relation thereto is constituted, partly the precipitate of all human experience pertaining to the opposite sex...The soul image is a more or less firmly constituted functional complex and the inability to distinguish one's self from it leads to such phenomena as those of the moody man, dominated by feminine drives, ruled by his emotions, or of the rationalizing, animus-obsessed woman who always knows better and reacts in a masculine way, not instinctively.

A will strange to us makes itself felt within us at certain times, which does the opposite of what we ourselves would want or approve. It is not necessarily that this other will does the evil; it also may will the better and be experienced then as a guiding or inspiring higher being, as a guardian spirit or genius in the sense of the Socratic "daimonion."[14]

Just as the anima is not merely a symbol and expression of the "snake," of the dangers of the drives waiting their chance for seduction in the dark of the unconscious but at the same time signifies man's light and inspiring guide, leading him onwards, not downwards, so is the animus not only the "devil of opinions," the renegade from all logic, but also a productive, creative being albeit not in the form of masculine productiveness but as fructifying work as "logos spermatikos." As the man gives birth to his work out of his inner femininity as a rounded whole and the anima thereby becomes his inspiring muse, so the inner masculinity of the woman often brings forth creative germs able to fertilize the feminine in the man...If the woman has once become conscious of this, if she knows how to deal with her unconscious and allows herself to be guided by her inner voice, then it will largely depend upon her whether she will be the "femme inspiratrice" or a rider of principles who always wants to have the last word, whether she will become the Beatrice or Xanthippe of the man.[15]

What, now does such a blending of the "shadow" with the "animus" or "anima" mean? When one disapproves of certain of one's qualities, the result is usually repression, rather than a patient acceptance of one's dark sides: to transform and outgrow them gradually by furthering the underdeveloped positive qualities.

By virtue of repression, the negative qualities persist and continue in the unconscious as the shadow; they may distort and poison the unconscious soul life by merging with and engulfing the heterosexual complementary personality which is destined to be the leading force of the soul in its evolution. The animus or anima which might be an impulse leading forward becomes an obsessive force, a fiendish tempter and seducer when "contaminated" with the shadow. In mythology, this psychic process appears described as Lucifer's fall from the heaven into the pit of the earth (the unconscious). The angel of light (consciousness, *Phosphor*), by virtue of his challenge and revolt against the evolution of man,[16] is transformed into the prince of darkness (the unconscious) and henceforth as Satan, the adversary and seducer, rules over fire and brimstone (*Sulphur:* sol—sun, ferre—to carry, actually denotes the shackled sun forces within the interior of the earth in volcanic activities, coal deposits, etc.). Thus, hell, the realm of *Sulphur,* is the unconscious psychic underworld,[17] which all too often is ruled not by the sun of the higher self[18] but by that part of our personality which, instead of being given the chance for expression and evolution of its problems, is held in scorn and repression. The psychological expression of the erupting "dark double" of *Sepia* thus is the complementary, heterosexual, psychic factor which by virtue of its suppression takes on a dark character; coalescing with the shadow, it appears as a negative and fiendish quality.†

Since, as outlined above, the repressive tendency of *Sepia* is directed particularly against the feminine character, its particular difficulty will be found more frequently in women with a rather masculine tendency; this fact is fully born out by clinical experience. Also a close functional relationship to *Sulphur* is to be expected from the above analysis of their psychic correlation.

As though nature wished to summarize the two main directions of the *Sepia* problem, namely towards the feminine per se, as represented by the oyster shell (Calc. carb.), and towards the psychological expression, as symbolized by the fiendish tempter or Satan (Sulfur), calcium salts and sulfur appear as the two main components of the melanin which makes up our *Sepia* clouds.[20, 21] Since melanin itself is an intermediary product of adrenalin formation, we are led to seek the physiologic aspect of the above psychological manifestations in disorders of the adrenal function. Endocrinology confirms our hypothesis and furnishes us with the key for the understanding of the correlated physical aspects of the pathology.

It is accepted that sex is determined by a preponderance of male or female producing genes in the combined chromosomes of sperm and ovum after fertilization; thus, even biologically, every person contains elements of the opposite sex. Even the hormones of ovaries and testes are not considered absolutely sex specific but are only stimulators of a preexistent sex character which is determined by the chromosomal structure. The total personality, as it were, determines sex. The gonads only execute or accentuate it.[22] While the gonads protect and intensify the preponderant disposition, the adrenal glands, on the other hand, promote the opposite, concealed sex character. The clinical condition called interrenalism (cortico-adrenal tumors) tends to produce feminism in men and masculinism in women. However, the female genetic structure seems to be more susceptible to this transmutation than the male one, since this transformation of the sex character is more frequent in women than in men.[23] This agrees with our finding from the psychological symbol interpretation that *Sepia's* "revolt" is against the feminine character. Also, clinically, we have found *Sepia* as a medicine more often indicated in women than in men.

Whereas an unbalanced hyperadrenalism of moderate sub-clinical degree probably underlies the heterosexual traits and the aggressiveness of the *Sepia* character (adrenal as the "gland of aggression"), the underfunction of the adrenals accounts for the asthenia, general ptosis, neurasthenia, hypotension and overpigmentation (melanosis). Those most characteristic features of the *Sepia* patient are milder manifestations of what, as gross pathology, appears in Addison's disease.

The dynamic formative principle underlying the unitarian totality of *Sepia* thus reveals itself as basically not uniform but very complex and characterized by inner tensions and contradictions. Its mental and physical symptomatology results from the participation in what we called the sphere of creativeness (oyster, *Calcarea,* femininity) and light (luminescence, like *Phosphor*) from the peculiar antithetic dynamism of the shadow and darkness, linking it to the *Sulphur* sphere as well as to the heterosexual personality complexes and of what we called the "masculine protest."

We now are able to explain the more detailed symptomatology as brought out in the provings.[24]

The mental symptoms are the outgrowth of the resented or repressed sexual role and of the eruption of the unconscious personality, the amalgamation of animus and shadow. This state of "being beside oneself" is complemented by the hypersensitivity of the disturbed light dynamism, similar to the state which we found in *Phosphor.*[25]

Thus the Materia Medica describes the *Sepia* patients as extremely *passionate, irritable, hysterical, full of tears* and *self pity; spiteful, antagonistic, faultfinding; never happy unless annoying someone, particularly those loved best; vexed at trifles; sad one minute, gentle and yielding the next; unable to give love and affection; averse to the opposite sex; greedy, miserly* and *egotistical; intolerant of opposition; oversensitive and easily offended; full of anxieties* and *fears (of darkness, illness, misfortune, being alone).* Like *Phosphor* they have states of *reverie, ecstasy* and *dreaminess.* The drive for individuality and self-expression which underlies the basic contradictory attitude is expressed in the *aversions* to *sympathy, consolation,* and *company;* and in the extremes of separativeness, aversion even to *one's family (husband, children)* and those who are *usually loved best.*

Of the physical symptoms we first turn to those which are accounted for by the disturbed light-darkness balance, manifesting itself through the adrenals. The influence of the adrenal dysfunction upon pigmentation and the ageing process gives a typical external aspect to the *Sepia* patient: *rigid fibre, sallow complexion, yellow freckles, loss of hair, early graying* and *premature ageing.* The colour of the hair, in particular, tends to be of an unusual or unexpected hue in adrenal types, e.g., blond in Italians or black in Norwegians and often is reddish.[26] Thus the fact is explained that in the homeopathic literature the "typical" *Sepia* patient has been described by turns as *dark haired, red haired,* or *blond* by different authors. Probably, each author was struck by the particular, in his instance, unusual hair colour which he described as the typical one.

Symptoms of hypoadrenalism are the *adynamia, indifference, indolence*, and *melancholic depression* which spring from vital exhaustion and tiredness in *Sepia*. Into the same category belong the *inability of mental concentration* and *dizziness* and *faintness.* In hypoadrenalism the general muscular tonus is reduced, thus bringing about a constitutional hypotension and *generalized ptosis (worse standing, lifting; involuntary urination upon coughing; low backache, prolapse, etc.).*

The hyperfunction of the adrenals with its heterosexual tendency combines with the disorder of the sex sphere which is the expression of the antifeminine attitude. Thus *Sepia* patients are often *masculine women* with *narrow pelves, overgrowth of body hair, tendency to beard and mustache* and *deep voice.* Men who need *Sepia* are quite often overly dry, rigid and hardened, less frequently the effeminate types of males, as with *Pulsatilla.* As the negation to the role of the woman extends itself to include the refusal of the role of the mother we find *homosexuality, sexual frigidity, aversion to the opposite sex* and *to husband and children.* The wide range of genital disorders, which includes almost every and any disturbance of menstruation, cohabitation, pregnancy and childbirth with their after effects, needs no further detailed elaboration. In the aggravation every 28 days we readily recognize the rhythm of the estric cycle.

Sepia's participation in the oyster-Calcarea family is expressed in a tendency to formlessness and a lack of resistance. The patient is *puffed, flabby, slow and indolent,* of a *soft, placid, mild, easy,* even *lazy disposition, incapable of any exertion;* "lymphatic"; "scrophulous" types or, as we call it now, suffering from an exudative, allergic diathesis with a dendency to *asthma, hayfever, urticaria, food allergies (worse strawberries, milk); sensitivity to cold air, lacking resistance against colds,* and venereal infections.

The antithesis, again, of the quiet *Calcarea* principle is found in the general, almost obsessive, restlessness and *amelioration from vigorous motion* and the *general erethismus* with *flashes of heat.* Also, the extreme tendency to *spasticity* with *globus* and *"ball"* sensations in various parts is explained by the suppression of the psychic and sexual impulses.

With *Phosphor*, the light carrier, *Sepia* shares the *aggravation in the afternoon, evening* and *before thunderstorms,* the *fear of being alone,* the *amelioration from eating and cold drinks* and the *affinity* for the *left* (unconscious) *side, as well* as the *lack of stamina* and the tendency to anemia.

Like *Phosphor* and *Sulphur,* we have a *hypersensitivity to odors* and a *desire for stimulating food.*

The subtle shades of difference in these last mentioned hypersensitivities are noteworthy since they shed a light on the universality of the formative idea inherent in the metamorphosis of the drug personality.

Sulphur's hypersensitivity is against body odors, the result of a faulty body and heat metabolism; *Phosphor's* is against the odor of flowers and perfumes, namely the end products of the heatless light metabolism of plants. Actually, the smell of flowers which promotes pollination by attracting insects corresponds to the body odor of animals which performs an equally attractive function as sexual odor (thus the role of perfumes and flowers in courtship and romance). In eating and digesting, the plant substance is transferred into the animal substance. Thus, eating and digesting (also cooking) are processes of predigestion, that carry over the plant (light) into the animal (heat) metabolism. *Sepia,* which integrates the *Phosphor* light with the fire-darkness of *Sulphur,* is *oversensitive* to the *odor of food.*

We find a similar situation in respect to food preferences. The highly seasoned, spicy foods which *Sulphur* craves are popularly called "hot" foods; they are prevalent in Southern hot climates where people also have "hot" temperaments. The stimulative effect of their ethereal oils is primarily upon the digestive processes. The salty food of the *Phosphor* craving awakens mind and consciousness (salt herring for the morning after; proverbially, "to take it with a grain of salt," meaning with careful deliberation). Salty foods are prevalent in the more deliberate and intellectual, colder northern countries. The sour taste which is craved by *Sepia,* in comparison, appears of a more emotional nature (compare "sourpuss," "surface" and the German saying: to give him "sour," meaning to upset his feelings).

The state of general ptosis, to a particular extent, makes itself felt in a slowing down of the *abdominal venous* circulation. We find *abdominal plethora* with *portal* and *pelvic congestion* resulting in a *tendency to hemorrhoids* and *varicose veins; bilious* and *dyspeptic disorders* with a *hypersensitivity* to fats and *intolerance to the pressure of clothes,* particularly around the waist. The systemic effects of *hepatic* stasis are *rheumatic* and *gouty disorders* with the *thick offensive urine* of high

102

specific gravity with *adherent red sediment* (probably phosphates and uric acid).

Inasmuch as the pull of gravity increases the venous engorgement, *standing aggravates* while lying down gives comparative relief. On the other hand, since exercise stimulates the circulation while rest encourages statis, we also find the opposite modalities of better from *vigorous exercise* and *worse* from *rest,* worse *during* and *after sleep.*

The general venous stasis with incomplete oxidation and elimination *Sepia* shares with the complementary *Sulphur.* Thus we can account for the *desire for fresh air* and the *lack of vital heat* (insufficient metabolic compensatory heat production) as well as for the disturbed skin function manifesting itself as *increased perspiration* and the wide array of dermatological disorders with the *Sulphur* modality of *worse from washing and bathing* (fire and water do not mix).

Also the respiratory symptoms are of a predominantly congestive nature as the result of stasis *(hypostatic pleuritis, cough apparently coming from the stomach, with a rather egg-like taste, worse evening and at night after sleep, better from rapid motion).* The *tubercular diathesis* is part of the *Calcarea* and *Phosphor* dynamism inherent in *Sepia.*

The technique which was used for the interpretation of the pathogenesis of a drug is in many respects similar to the way in which analytical psychology unravels the symbolic context of the unconscious material of patients as found in dreams, visions and associations. In succeeding in the "analysis" of a drug we bear out the hypothesis of a probably identical basic entity underlying the different levels of manifestation in symbol formation, morphology and psychologic, as well as biologic, evolution. The creative spirit in nature, as well as in man, expresses itself through the metamorphosis of basic archetypes.

"In the fact that that which is of similar concept may appear in its manifestations as like or similar, yet even as totally unlike and dissimilar, in this fact consists the ever changing life of nature."[27]

---

[1]Jung, C.G. *Collected Works* 12 *(Psychology and Alchemy,* NY 1953), p. 170-71.
[2]*Ibid.,* pp. 84, 147.
[3]*Ibid.,* pp. 170-71, 225-28.
[4]*Ibid.,* pp. 143 ff.
[5]Wilhelm Reich, *The Function of the Orgasm* (New York, Orgone Institute Press, 1942), pp. 232, 240 ff., 257 ff., 269.
[6]Edward Whitmont, Natrum muriaticum, *The Homeopathic Recorder,* LXIII:5: 188 ff. (Nov., 1947).

[7]David Tomtsett, Sepia *Publ. Liverpool Marine Biolog. Committee, Memories* No. 32 (Liverpool, University Press, Sept., 1939), pp. 144, 145.

[8]William Gutman, Sepia, *Journal of the American Institute of Homeopathy,* 36:12:438 ff. (December, 1943).

[9]Karl Dominicus, *Homeop. Arzneimittelpruefung am Gesunden Menschen mit Sepia* (Paderborn, Bonifaciusdruckerei, 1937), p. 11.

[10]Edward Whitmont, Phosphor, *The Homeopathic Recorder,* LXIV:10:258 ff. (April, 1949).

[11]Jung, C.G. *Collected Works* 12, pp. 143ff.

[12]Edward Whitmont, Towards a Basic Law of Psychic and Somatic Inter-relationship, *The Homeopathic Recorder,* LXV:8:202FF. (Feb., 1950).

[13]Carl G. Jung, *The Integration of the Personality* (New York, Toronto, Farrar and Rinehart, Inc. 1939) pp. 18-21. Rearranged by permission of Bollingen Foundation, N.Y.

[14]Jolan Jacobi, *The Psychology of Jung* (New Haven; Yale University Press, 1943), pp. 104ff.

[15]*Ibid,* pp. 104ff.

[16]*Ibid.,* pp. 109ff.

[17]*The Apocryphal New Testament.* The Bible of the World, edit. by Rob. Q. Balon (New York, The Viking Press, 1939) pp. 1272, 1273.

[18]Jung, C.G. *Collected Works* 12 (*Psychology and Alchemy,* N. Y. 1953), pp. 315ff.

[19]Carl G. Jung, *The Integration of the Personality,* New York, Toronto, Farrar and Rinehart, 1939), p. 122.

[20]William Gutman, Sepia, *Journal of the American Institute of Homeopathy,* 36:12:438ff. (December, 1943).

[21]Karl Dominicus, *Homeop. Arzneimittelpruefung am Gesunden Menschen mit Sepia* (Paderborn, Bonifaciusdruckerei, 1937), p. 11.

[22]Julius Bauer, *Constitution and Disease* (New York, Grune & Stratton, 1945), pp. 82, 83.

[23]*Ibid,* pp. 86, 87.

[24]Symptoms quoted directly from provings and listed in the homeopathic *Materia Medica,*(Kent, hering, Clarke, etc.) are in italics.—E.W.

[25]Edward Whitmont, Phosphor, *The Homeopathic Recorder,* LXIV:10:258ff. (April, 1949).

[26]Louis Berman, *The Glands Regulating Personality* (New York, Macmillan, 1928), p. 237.

[27]Johann Wolfgang V. Goethe, *Morphologie* (Stuttgart, Collected Works, J.G. Cotta, Ed., 1874) Vol. 14, p. 5.

†The peculiar quality of the devilish tempter and seducer, appearing in the vestments of the opposite sex, we find expressed as psychological entities in the "succubi" and "incubi" of the Middle Ages.

PHOSPHOR

Phosphor, in its active yellow form, exhibits a phenomenon which is unique among the non-radioactive substances. It produces *light without heat independently of any exogenous irradiation.* This luminescence is not incidental to a disintegration of the particles of matter but to the *synthesis of a more complex compound, the oxide.* Whereas the disintegration-products of radioactivity are rather inimical to vital functioning, the oxidation products of *Phosphor* are more closely related to the living process. They participate actively in metabolism and cell structure. Unlike radioactivity, the *Phosphor* luminescence appears positively integrated into the cycles of life-functioning.

The oxidation of *Phosphor* is furthermore characterized by its gradual and slow pace. Rapid oxidation leads to loss of luminescence by rapid consumption in burning, while heat without oxygen abolishes the luminescence by converting the yellow phosphorus into the red, inactive modification. Thus, even in the most elementary form, the light activity is distinctly defined as different from heat processes.

Within the living organism the luminescence of ingested material can still be demonstrated, even after days, by the Mitscherlich process as used in forensic medicine. In spite of being exposed to the tremendous oxidizing power of the blood, *Phosphor* thus maintains its own independent autonomous rhythm within the organism.[1] We are justified in assuming that what is so readily demonstrated in the gross, material process would not necessarily be abolished in the finer state of colloidal dispersion where, as yet, we lack means for direct identification. Moreover, what is a physical phenomenon in the crude substance becomes a dynamic tendency in the potentized intramolecular functioning, the probable basis for all coordinated life-functioning.

A preliminary hypothesis of an autonomous 'inner light' regulation or metabolism, analogous to the autonomous inner heat regulation suggests itself. Just as the autonomous heat regulation depends upon the variations of outer warmth, so may the regulation of our 'inner light' depend upon the interplay with outer light, yet be self-regulating in its own sphere.†

In order to test the validity of this hypothesis our first step will be a survey of what is known about the function of light in relation to our psychosomatic unit.

We may note the interesting fact that the word *'Phosphor',* translated from the Greek, means 'carrier', or *'conveyor of light'.* The identical meaning is encountered in the Latin word, 'Lucifer', Phosphor-Lucifer is the angel who *rebelled against the Godhead and conveyed the light of reasoning to men so that they 'shall be as gods, knowing good and evil.'* (Gen. 3:5)

Jung has shown that the symbolism of language, mythology and alchemy express a genuine intuitive awareness of unconscious but nevertheless quite actual dynamics of psyche and cosmos. The treasure of wisdom inherent in such material far transcends what slow evidence our gradual conscious research has been able to gather. None of it need be accepted at face value, but it may indicate new directions for research which will enrich our knowledge providing we can find confirmatory evidence. The practice of analytical psychology has repeatedly verified that evidence in its own field and in psychosomatics.

The symbolic significance of *light,* as a transcendental force-principle, represents the *'inner spiritual man',*[2] and the qualities of *consciousness, wisdom and intellect.*[3,4] Darkness stands for the realm of the unconscious psyche.[5] Of particular interest to us is the concept of the 'dark light', which appears in an alchemistic source and would be analogous to our postulated invisible, internal light activity of *Phosphor.* In this alchemistic 'dark light' we can discover a similarity to the light that 'shineth in the darkness; and the darkness comprehended it not' (St. John 1:5). As a matter of fact, in this alchemistic source the 'dark light', as inner light, is identified with the 'monogenes' which means the 'only begotten one',[6] the 'Son of Man', the 'Light of the World'. Thus the inner light, as a conceptual mental entity in the image of Lucifer, the materialistic intellect,[7] arouses men from a state of *childlike, paradisical, unconscious innocence and exalts itself in the 'Son of Man' to represent the highest and sublimest force-principle of universal and personal consciousness.*

Upon further scrutiny of the symbol material we encounter the principle of inner light as 'logos' or 'nous' (intelligence or awareness) identified with 'pneuma',[8] meaning spirit, but also breath. Thus Adam, of whom the book of Genesis records that "God breathed into his nostrils the breath of life; and man became a living soul" (Genesis 2:7), has in gnosis the given name of 'light'[9] which is to indicate his inner spiritual entity.[10] Lucifer, the representative of the intellect, is depicted as an air spirit.[11]

Another mythological representation of the light-carrier is Prometheus who, according to the Greek legend, seized the fire from the heavens for man and was bound by Zeus to Mt. Caucasus to have a vulture daily consume his liver. Prometheus, whose name literally translated means 'forthinker', is also called the 'light man' or 'inner man'[12] in the gnosis. The vulture who devours his physical liver again depicts thought and intellectualism.[13]

In Steiner's anthroposophical system *Phosphor* is likened to the tendencies which are sublimating, dissolving and etherizing as contrasted to the concentrating, crystallising tendencies expressed by Sal. Also here, *Phosphor* is associated with light, as a dynamic principle to be found everywhere in nature. In the plant, for instance, Sal represents the root, *Phosphor* the blossom.

Jung also refers to the blossom as the symbol of the spiritual self,[14] thus confirming the uniformity, throughout, of the meaning of the Phosphor-light symbol as the representation of spiritual consciousness.

To summarize, we may state that the force-principle, called *Phosphor, has to do with inner spiritual light, insight, intellect and ego-control. As flower, it reflects the spirit of the spheres, refining and etherizing.* As 'pneuma', it expresses itself in *breath or respiration* (Homer still has his heroes think in their diaphragm) and, as *vulture, it destroys the liver.* The main directions of the clinical *Phosphor* effects already stand out. It remains to be seen if these inspired 'phantasies' can prove useful to the understanding and ordering of the available clinical and experimental evidence, and help us to explain hitherto unexplainable facts.

We turn now to the biologic effects of light.

Plants kept in complete darkness do not grow. A small, insufficient amount of light produces stooping or creeping overgrowth; an excess of substance is produced at the expense of stamina and color (compare mushroom and fungus growth). Conversely, mountain and desert plants, exposed to a super abundance of light, develop extremely short but sturdy stems (even when sheltered from wind) with particularly bright, beautifully colored blossoms.

In the animal organism, strongly growing, embryonal organs have an increased radiosensitivity.[15] Purely vegetative growth is sensitive to over-radiation.

On the human organism the effect of light is described as generally vitalizing and strengthening, stimulating *perception* and the *ability to think.* Finsen especially stresses the fact that this effect is not merely psychological but takes place on the biochemical level.[16] So profound and basic is this awakening effect that it abolishes the soporific, *depressing, central nervous effect of anesthetics and intoxicants;* in order to induce anesthesia in high altitude, a greater concentration of anesthetic is required, not only in the alveolar air (which could be explained as due to the lessened air pressure), but in the bloodstream itself. A greater awareness of the nerve centers has to be overcome. Similarly, a higher concentration of alcohol is required in the bloodstream to cause intoxication.[17] A basic antagonism is indicated here between *light and the consciousness-depressing effect of anesthetics* and alcohol; this antagonism appears not limited to the functional sphere only, but affects also the organic physiologic level. The fact that *light stabilizes an overexcited nervous system* points in the same direction (excitation is similar to the primary effect of alcohol and anesthetics). The *sympathicus tonus is reduced* and the *blood pressure decreased.*[18]

Thyroid disturbances are favorably affected.[19]

An analogy to the increase of stamina and firmness in plants can be found in the skeletal effects of light. *It prevents and cures rickets and promotes the healing of bone fractures,* as well as of *wounds in general.* In Swiss experiments a marked statistical difference is shown between patients in well-lighted rooms and those in darker rooms in the time required for the union of bone fractures.[20]

Light increases the blood calcium level, stimulates motor activity and circulation, favorably affects the coronaries, and raises the minute volume of the heart. The erythrocyte count is increased.[21]

Finally, there is a definite effect upon the respiratory system: *Light increases the ventilation of the lungs and the depth of breathing.*[22] *Pulmonary tuberculosis is favorably affected by small amounts, yet extremely sensitive to strong light radiation,* while the nonpulmonary Tb. responds favorably to any degree of radiation[23] (here we already may note the close similarity to the sensitivity to *Phosphor* dosage). Trivial respiratory infections *vanish most rapidly in the intense radiation of high altitudes.*

There is a general *anti-infectious effect* of light which is probably due to *increased resistance as well as to anti-bacterial action.* Over-radiation on the other hand promotes local as well as general inflammatory response with increased protein breakdown and febrile reaction.

Summarizing, we have:

1. A mental direction of the light effects, in enhancing and stabilizing the functions of consciousness and in its antagonism to the action of anesthetics.

2. A general effect, regulating growth and enhancing general vitality and resistance, as well as the firmness of the physical structure.

These two, the mental and general, effects provide the key to the whole pathology, as we shall see, and determine the effects upon particular organs, namely the respiratory, circulatory and locomotor systems.

So far, this exposition of the light physiology seems already to agree surprisingly well with the main directions suggested by the symbolical meaning of light *as "nous," insight, and "pneuma," breath.*

How does all this relate to the more detailed symptomatology of *Phosphor?*

According to our hypothesis a normal state of *Phosphor*-functioning would consist in the *undisturbed action of the inner light.* Since a complete paralysis of this function, absolute darkness as it were, probably would be incompatible with life, we might liken the clinical *Phosphor* disturbance to a state of inner twilight. How would such a twilight state be expected to express itself?

In our analysis, we may well enough follow the classification arrived at in the summary of the light pathology:

1. Effect upon the consciousness as opposed to the effects of anesthetics and intoxicants.

The gradual ascendance of conscious and cerebral control represents a relatively recent achievement of the gradual evolution of man. When the full light of consciousness is weakened, impulses come to the fore which are normally relegated to the dark pool of the unconscious. A relapse occurs into earlier, more instinctual and imaginal states. Reactions like *clairvoyance*,[24] *clairaudience* or *ecstasy* may occur, *apparitions* may be seen, rationally unaccounted for and consequently disturbing and threatening to the patient *(fanciful and imaginary notions, faces grinning out of every corner, as if something would creep out of every corner, etc.)*.

When the borderline between the accustomed daily reality and the assumed "unreality" of the unconscious weakens, when the unconscious invades the upper stratum of conscious reality, the response is always one of *fear. Phosphor* has *fear of being alone,* since the presence of people helps to strengthen the accustomed reality against the invasion from the darker strata, *fear that something may happen, of death, fear of the darkness, of evening, night* and characteristically enough, of the *twilight* which is the outward projection of the inner psychological state and consequently accentuates and aggravates the total psychosomatic state.

However, the classical picture of what happens when the inner light acting in our moral consciousness is dimmed is provided experimentally by the observation of drunkenness and anesthesia. Here the conscious and cerebral control is removed and the individual allows himself to revert to a quasi-infantile state in which the instincts hold free sway. Light was found to be directly antagonistic to the action of alcohol and anesthetics. Moreover, the symptoms and organic changes caused by the aliphatic lipoid-soluble anesthetics (alcohol, ether and chloroform) which resemble one another in their main actions,[25] when considered together, show a most striking similarity to the *Phosphor* pathogenesis, thus suggesting the actual relevance of this material for our purpose (for brevity, alcohol, ether and chloroform, when not especially differentiated, will be reffered to simply as anesthetics.)

The effect of intoxication, which resembles also the beginning of anesthesia, is described as follows:[26]

It depresses the central nervous system, especially the higher functions. *It stimulates, chiefly by lowering the normal restraining functions* ...resulting in euphoria, comfort and

109

enjoyment, to elation and vivacity; then downward through loquacity, garrulity, emotionalism, either affectionate or quarrelsome or both, to violence, then hebetude, stupor and finally coma.

This pattern is most closely duplicated in the *Phosphor* pathogenesis. The provings show a polarity of *excitability and ecstasy* with lowered inhibitions followed by *indifference, stupor and exhaustion.* The *Phosphor* patient resembles the devotee of Bacchus in being *pleasant, sympathetic,* of *sanguine temperament, changeable disposition* or *quarrelsome* and *easily angered, craving company, loquacious, amative, easily enthused* but unreliable, without perseverance, *impressionable* and *very susceptible to external influences with quick perception, increased flow of thoughts* which *rush through his mind* (stimulative phase), subject to states of *mania of grandeur* yet quickly given to *exhaustion and fatigue* (depressive phase), *unable to stand mental tax, unable to think and worse from mental exertion,* becoming *hyposensitive, apathetic* and *indifferent* with *failing memory and concentration, aversion to work* ending in stupor and coma.

Emotionally the loss of inhibitions makes him *easily excited, getting beside himself with anger, vehement, perspiring from excitement* (as does the drinker and the anesthetized patient), *fearful, cowardly, sad hysterical, alternatingly laughing and crying,* or just *tearful* and gloomy, *weary of life,* and *misanthropic.*

The loss of moral inhibitions results in the ascendence of the more animalistic and indiscriminate impulses: *lasciviousness, uncovers his person, seeks to gratify his sex instincts no matter on whom, erotic mania, sex excitement and shamelessness.*

Obviously, the similarity between the *Phosphor* picture and anesthesia (the somatic sphere of which will be discussed later) holds therapeutic implications. *Mania-a-potu, delirium tremens, ill effects of ether and chloroform* and clinical *Phosphor* indications.

2. Effect on growth-regulation and general vitality and resistance.

The lack of stamina within the mental personality is paralleled by a loss of stamina in the physical sphere. We may compare this with the analogous disturbance of plants with insufficient light exposure. Such plants show overgrowth, with long, stooping, pale, weakly stems, or the abundant over-production of soft material as found in mushrooms and fungi. Extremest light privation, of course, leads to stunted growth.

The materia medica of *Phosphor* lists: *Feeble constitutions, born sick, grown up slender, young people who grow too rapidly, stooping, bad posture, stunted growth; chlorotic girls who grow too rapidly and have suddenly taken on weakness, pallor and green sickness* (Kent). The failure to form chlorophyll in the pale, lightless plants or mushrooms has its counterpart in the deficient formation of hemoglobin; moreover we remember that light increases the red cell count. *Anemia* thus becomes an obvious finding in a state of disturbed light-functioning. In analogy to the lack of the generally vitalizing effect of light, the inner twilight state of *Phosphor* has the typical *adynamia; mentally and physically exhausted, always tired, need of rest; easily weakened by loss of vital fluids, empty, all gone sensation in chest (the chest, the seat of the "pneuma,"* being particularly under the light-Phosphor influence), *lack of vital heat.* The exhaustion which follows the mental overexcitation (see above) is augmented by this constitutional physical lack of resilience. *Emaciation* and *marasmus* are the final states of the extreme mental and physical exhaustion.

Progressive adynamia is commonly associated with failure of the *adrenal glands, and, actually, Phosphor poisoning depresses the adrenals.*[27] In turn we are led to assume a close association of the adrenals to our postulated inner light-metabolism by the fact that they regulate the formation of melanin, the dark pigment in the skin, hair, retina, etc., which is the organism's response to light. The *Phosphor* type with its lessened light activity and reduced adrenal functioning is more often found to be *blond, soft haired* (also, the hair growth, as such, is under adrenal control) and *light-complexioned.*

The adrenal disturbance also explains the circulatory and cardiac weakness with lowered sympathicus tonus (adrenalin is the sympathicus hormone), as well as the peculiar modality of the *craving for salt* (Addison's disease has sometimes been favorably affected by massive salt doses).

While younger people furnish the analogy to the over-grown stooping plant, the fungus- or mushroom-like tendency of abounding growth is found where a longitudinal expansion no longer is possible. Since the normal channel of growth is blocked, the dammed up tendency expresses itself in tumor growth. It is not by chance that tumor cells resemble embryonal cells and that both have an increased radiosensitivity[28] as the expression of a more precarious light balance. The pathogenesis of *Phosphor* includes *cancer* and *fibroids.*

The personality described so far, devoid of mental firmness as well as of vital stamina, is bound to be a drifting straw, an almost helpless victim of outer influences and inner emotions. The provings account for this by eliciting *oversensitivity* to almost any outer and inner factor (viz., *light, noise, odors, touch, electricity, thunderstorms, changing weather, dampness, etc.; mind too impressionable, excitable, etc.*)

Finding no source of strength within himself, he must look for support and recharging of his energies from without, thus always depending and leaning upon others: *desire for company, fear of being alone, desire for and better from rubbing, massaging and mesmerization.*

111

When the symptoms are confined only to potential tendencies, rather than the extremer manifestations which we described, the average well-known *Phosphor* type results:

A sociable sympathetic, pleasant person of rather sanguine temperament, very adaptable, enthusiastic but unreliable, with but little perseverance and strength of character, drifting with the current; probably quite artistic, given to day dreaming and romance, sensitive and easily influenced; he looks tall, slender, narrow chested with fair, transparent skin, soft hair and delicate eyelashes, is easily exhausted and has but little physical strength and staying power. He is oversensitive to the "vibrations" of others and incidentally also to drugs, both crude and potentised.

All in all he is a truly flower- or butterfly-like being, thriving in the sunshine of favorable circumstances but wilting in the darkness and coldness of adversity.

If we contrast this *Phosphor* blossom with the slow, steady, persevering, introverted *Natrum mur.* type which typifies the alchemistic 'sal', or root principle, we have an impressive example of the deep intuitive insight into the secret workings of nature as expressed in this symbol terminology.

The remaining 'particulars', symptoms referred to specific organs, unfold themselves out of the same two main directions of light:

A. The mental effect upon consciousness as opposed by anesthetics leads to the action upon the

    1. Nervous and muscular systems and lipoid metabolism

    2. Digestive system

    3. Circulation and respiration

    4. Oxidation mechanism

B. The general effect upon growth, general resistance and stamina explains the action of *Phosphor* upon the skeleton and the calcium metabolism.

The close similarity between the mental symptoms of *Phosphorus* and the lipoid-soluble anesthetics, which, as we shall see, is paralleled by almost identical physical effects, signifies a fundamental basic correlation between *Phosphor* and the anesthetics. We are entitled to the conclusion that those physical symptoms which are common to both of them, express the organic changes which result from a reduced state of consciousness and ego-control, the weakened inner "light man."

1. *Anesthetics paralyze the central nervous system by virtue of their lipoid affinity and solubility.* Apparently, as one result of this *selective lipoid toxicity, lipoid and fat infiltration occurs in various organs (liver, heart, muscle, etc.)*

The lipoid affinity of *Phosphor* is well enough known: *Phosphor* occurs in the serum almost exclusively in the form of phosphor lipoids,[29] which are considered important structural as well as functional elements of the nervous system. Subsequent to the loss of control of the higher centers, as described, organic nervous disorders will occur as the result of the disturbance of the lipoid metabolism. The modality, *worse from rising,* finds its explanation in the fact that in the upright (awake) position the conscious cerebral control is supposed to prevail, while the horizontal position corresponds to the function of lower centers during sleep as well as to the animalic (with horizontal spine), instinctive level. The many organic nervous symptoms need not be enumerated here in detail.

Also, the muscular apparatus with its close functional association to nerve and bone (see later) will participate in the *Phosphor*-induced disturbance (the muscle function depends upon hexose phosphoric acid as intermediary product for its function.)

The lipoid infiltration of anesthetics is duplicated in the fatty degeneration of liver, heart and other organs which occurs in *Phosphor* poisoning. Of special interest to us is a symptom consisting of muscle degeneration with simultaneous fat infiltration, the *muscular pseudo-hypertropy,* a leading clinical *Phosphor* indication.

It is of interest to remember that the childhood state is characterized *by a relative abundance of fat deposits.* Mentally and emotionally, the child, with its undeveloped sense of responsibility and ego-control, seems to represent a quasi-physiological *Phosphor* state (growing organisms, of course, are particularly sensitive to *Phosphor* instabilities merely by virtue of their growing). The tendency to fat deposits, shared alike by child and chronic alcoholic, thus presents itself as a characteristic somatic feature of the childish, careless frame of mind. We may recall the intuitive recognition of this fact in art, as expressed in the immortal Falstaff, and Caesar's words: "Let me have men about me that are fat..." (Shakespeare, *Julius Caesar,* Act 1, Scene II).

2. *Anesthetics cause gastrointestinal irritation* (alcoholic gastritis, nausea and vomiting of alcohol, ether, chloroform). *Phosphor* shows a correspondingly similar irritative tendency leading to its long list of clinical indications of this sphere. Of special interest to us are the modalities of the *craving for salt and spices* and the *desire for ice-cold water which is vomited as soon as it gets warm in the stomach.* These symptoms of *Phosphor* are quite characteristic for the disturbance of the drinker, as well (salt herring for the morning after, etc.). An empty stomach makes us light-headed and faint, eating restores us to ourselves. Similarly, eating counteracts the effects of intoxicating spirits and the light-headed *Phosphor* patient is *better from eating.*

The similarity between the Phosphor hepatitis and the acute yellow atrophy with fat infiltration of the chloroform liver has been referred to already. Moreover, *Phosphor* causes liver cirrhosis,[30] *thus parelleling the cirrhosis of alcohol.* Recently, this alcohol cirrhosis has been associated with a protein deficiency: *Phosphor* poisoning which leads to an increased loss due to breakdown of the protein[31] bears out even this detail.

The intimate relationship between liver function and *synthesis of Vitamin K and fibrinogen,* along with the influence of the *disturbed* calcium balance (see later), explain the hemorrhagic tendency of *Phosphor* which is duplicated again by ether.[32]

Anesthetics cause hyperglycemia and glycosuria.[33] So does *Phosphor* by inhibiting the synthesis of glycogen in the liver.[34] Diabetes frequently occurs in constitutional types who appear not firmly rooted within themselves but are of a rather soft, dreamy type, very susceptible to the disintegrating effect of emotional shocks which so often were found to have caused diabetes.

Thus the general metabolic effect of *Phosphor* fits into the pattern of the disturbed or, if we use our symbol picture, *shackled 'light man' who suffers the vulture daily to destroy the liver.*

3. *Anesthetics impair the respiratory and circulatory apparatus: bronchitis, pneumonia of ether, heart failure of chloroform,* fatty heart of alcohol, chronic alcoholism predisposing to pneumonia.[35] *Phosphor,* likewise, is one of the outstanding remedies in those very conditions. The paramount position of the respiratory and, to a somewhat lesser extent, of the circulatory sphere within the pathogenesis of *Phosphor* and anesthetics draws our attention again to the equivalence of 'nous' and 'pneuma', mind and breath. Yet, how, exactly, would our consciousness reflect itself in our physical breathing? Since the question probably never arose in any research work, only few facts are available to us for attempting an answer. Respiration and pulse rate differ during sleep and wakefulness, but also during a state of strained attention. Forced overventilation produces tetany, not unlike the convulsive state caused by overdoses of stimulants (tetrazol). *It is well known that breath control and breathing affect consciousness.*

Breathing and circulation as active functions arise first at the very point of evolution which is characterized by the transition of the merely living, soulless plant to the perceiving animal. Breathing appears to be nearer to our conscious functioning than circulation which responds more to emotional impulses (all respiratory muscles are subject to voluntary innervation). This is in accord with the fact that in the development of the species as well as of the individual (biogenetic law) a circulation is established long before lung breathing appears. Thus the lung breathing actually seems to be related to an evolutionary, *relatively further advanced level of mental development.*

Light which enhances consciousness was also found to strengthen the respiratory system.

For a full explanation we are still at loss. However, these facts may make us less unwilling to take into serious consideration for further research the likelihood, at least, of the association of mind and breath, "nous" and "pneuma," as two phases of the metamorphosis of the light principle.

4. *Anesthetics lower the oxygen consumption of the tissue cells, poisoning resulting in oxygen starvation. Phosphor* seems to have a balancing or gently stimulating effect upon cellular oxidation analogous to the slow, but steady in vitro oxidation which maintains its luminescence (larger doses paralyse, small *Phosphor* doses stimulate cellular oxidation[36]). A bridge is thrown to the disturbed growth process by the fact that tumor tissue is characterized by lessened cellular respiration. *Phosphor, when curative in tumor cases, would thus change the anoxybiotic respiration of the tumor cells back to the normal oxybiotic type.*

A correlation may exist between this anoxybiotic type of cell metabolism and the increased protein breakdown which is common to toxic doses of light, anesthetics, and *Phosphor.*[37] As the bloodstream becomes overloaded with the toxic intermediary metabolic products, the *tendency to fevers, infections* and *septic states* arises. The protein loss accounts for the clinical symptom of *emaciation.* The more permanent, chronic, constitutional state of this type is found in the *phthisical, consumptive* condition.

5. Very revealing is the fact that ether or chloroform hasten the *blooming of flowers.*[38] A stimulative action reveals its selective affinity to just the blossom part of the plant. As outlined before, the alchemistic term, *Phosphor,* refers to the etherizing tendency expressed in the blossom; in our characterisation of the *Phosphor* personality we were led to liken him to a blossom or butterfly, because of his delicate over-refinement and lightness. Of the whole plant, the blossom part shows the greatest dependence upon light as revealed in its response with colors. Moreover, the blossom, when intensified in fragrance and perfumes, exhibits a somewhat narcotic tendency itself, mildly *benumbing to the mind and stimulative to the sexual instincts.* Characteristically, the *Phosphor* patient is *over-sensitive to and aggravated by the odor of flowers and perfumes* which strike an over-responsive chord in him.

B. Growth and firmness of the physical frame are reflected in the condition of the osseous skeleton; the calcium metabolism shows a close physiological interdependence with *Phosphor.*

Light activates ergosterol (which characteristically is also a member of the lipoid family) *into Vitamin D, the antirachitic factor. Lack of light causes not only rickets but also lowers the resistance against infections and predisposes to tuberculosis.* The dependence of bone repair and wound healing upon light was referred to before. The wide range of *Phosphor* indications in disorders of the skeleton (rickets, osteoporosis, osteomyelitis, osseous tuberculosis, etc.) requires no further elaboration.

The nature of the association of *Calcium* with *Phosphorus* deserves our attention, however. A parallelism seems to exist between calcification and firmness of the skeletal frame and a properly evolving mind. *Calcium deficiency reduces the ability for mental performance, and experimentally causes stupidity.* In sections with endemic osteomalacia there is a higher incidence of mental disorders during pregnancy which so greatly increases the *Calcium* deficiency with osteoporosis is a common finding.[39] Late closure of the fontanelles and rickets are often associated with slower mental development (in these cases *Phosphor,* like *Calcium,* will have a special *affinity to the bones of the skull).* The transition from childhood to adult life with its mental maturity is marked by completed calcification and epiphyseal closure. *The pseudo-infantile state of old age, again,* has a tendency to osteoporosis.

Thus the *proper firmness and integration of the physical frame appear to be paramount factors upon which a mental development is conditioned.* It becomes understandable that the force-principle of light, commissioned, as it were, with the task of developing our ego, consciousness and personal responsibility also must be concerned with the solidification of the physical frame which is to be the vehicle and instrument of our mind.

An energy complex which encompasses the very forces of personality with the vital and regenerative abilities, the resistance to infections, liver function and protein metabolism, as well as the bones themselves, cannot fail to have a most profound influence upon the very essence of our life, the blood. Light increases the red cell count; over-radiation of the higher wave length (X ray) profoundly disturbs the bone marrow. The *Phosphor* pathogenesis includes *anemia,* as well as *polycythemia, hemorrhagic* and *hemolytic* conditions, as well as *leucemia.*

Before closing we should consider one more important general modality. The *Phosphor* illness shows an outspokenly selective tendency to the *left side.* We know that the function of the two different sides is deeply interwoven with problems of the total personality (mental problems of lefthandedness) and the action of brain centers.

For the average righthanded individual the whole right side of his body is under much more conscious nerve control, innervated by the left, the rational and intellectual brain hemisphere.

The paramount general reality of this fact is confirmed by the analytic symbol-interpretation and has found its expression even in the often intuitive understanding of our language. Left symbolizes the unconscious,[40] and therefore is the sinister (Latin sinistra, threatening evil) side. The opposite is the "right" (good, correct) one because it is representative of our conscious actions.

Since the stage of our activities is also the battlefield upon which we receive our (often self-inflicted) wounds, the more active side seems also to be the side more liable to pathology. Thus the illness which emerges from the psychosomatic totality of an overintellectual and overconscientious *Lycopodium* type is rightsided, while the *Phosphor* sufferer, who has reverted to the more instinctive unconscious levels in his psychophysical expressions, presents us with leftsided pathology.

Based on the hypothetical assumption of an inner autonomous light regulation or light metabolism, we have set out to investigate the available material in its relation to the pathogenesis of *Phosphorus*. The interpretation of the symbol material as presented by the analytical psychology of Jung has offered us the suggestion to seek in this material the expression of a metamorphosis of the dynamic principle of light, manifesting in the forces of the higher personality, through intellect and breath down to the function of liver and metabolic organs. It furnished the framework into which we fitted our material evidence. Much of the hitherto disconnected material of mental and physical symptoms and modalities along with experimental, toxicologic and clinical features has thereby revealed a logical coherence as parts of one basic, immanent pattern. By circumstantial evidence, as it were, we have also confirmed the probably correctness of our assumption of an autonomous inner light balance, as well as the great informative value of the analytical symbol material.

---

[1]Hugo P.F. Schultz, Vorlesungen ueber Wirkung und Anwedung der unorganischen Arzneistoffe fuer Aertze und Studierende (Berlin, Karl F. Mang, 1939) pp. 125-6.

†The postulate of a light 'metabolism' where no light at all can be seen directly within the body may at first appear strange. Yet even this difficulty may resolve itself in view of recent discoveries concerning the regulation of physical functions by radiation-like phenomena arising within the organism. It may only be a limitation of our present techniques which prevents us from direct 'visualization' of such radiant microphenomena.—E.W.

[2]Jung, C.G. *Collected Works* 12 *(Psychology and Alchemy,* NY 1953), pp. 346-56.

[3]*Ibid.,* pp. 177-78; pp. 306-07.

[4]*CW* 13 *(Alchemical Studies,* Princeton 1967), p. 126.

[5]*CW* 12, pp. 315-17.

[6]*Ibid.*, p. 105.

[7]*Ibid.*, pp. 87-8.

[8]*Ibid.*, p. 289.

[9]*Ibid.*, p. 350.

[10]*Ibid.*, pg. 356.

[11]*Ibid.*, p. 88.

[12]*Ibid.*, pp. 350-52, p. 356.

[13]*Ibid.*, pp. 66, 128, 160-61, 193.

[14]*Ibid.*, p. 147.

[15]W. Hausman, Lichtbiologie und Lichtpathologie (Urban und Schwarzenberg, 1925), Sonderabdruck aus Lehrbuch der Strahlentherapie, Vol. 1, p. 631.

[16]N.R. Finsen, Die Bedutung der chemischen Strahlen des Lichtes (Leipzig, Vogel, 1899), pp. 58-64.

[17]A. Lowey, Die therapeutische Bedeutung des Hohenklimas, Transactions of the 7th Sportarztetagung in Meunchen, 1930, p. 62.

[18]*CW* 12, p. 289.

[19]A. Lowey, op. cit., p. 67.

[20]*Ibid.*, p. 64.

[21]W. Hausman, op. cit., p. 675.

[22]*Ibid.*, p. 671.

[23]A. Lowey, op. cit., p. 66.

[24]Symptoms directly quoted from the Homeopathic Materia Medica are in italics.

[25]Torald Sollman, Manual of Pharmacology (Philadeplia, W.B. Saunders Co., 1948), p. 603.

[26]*Ibid.*, p. 607.

[27]Otto Leeser, Textbook of Homeopathic Materia Medica, Inorganic Medicinal Substances (quoting Neubauer and Porges) (Philadelphia, Boericke and Tafel, 1935), p. 300.

[28]W. Hausman, Lichtbiologie und Lichtpathologie (Urban and Schwarzenberg, 1925), Sonderabdruck aus Lehrbuch der Strahlentherapie, Vol. 1, p. 631.

[29]Torald Sollman, op. cit., p. 646.

[30]*Ibid.*, p. 755.

[31]Hugo P. F. Schultz, op. cit., p. 646.

[32]Torald Sollman, op. cit., p. 646.

[33]*Ibid.*, p. 642.

[34]*Ibid.*, p. 756.

[35]*Ibid.*, p. 623.

[36]Otto Leeser, op. cit. (quoting Nishura), p. 300.

[37]Torald Sollman, op. cit., pp. 618, 756.

[38]*Ibid.*, p. 645.

[39]Oscar Loew, Der Kalkbedarf von Menschen und Tier (Muenchen, Verlag der aertzlichen Rundschau, O. Gmelin, 4th ed., 1927), pp. 33, 34.

[40]*CW* 12, pp. 121, 156, 163-64, 166, 177.

CALCAREA AND MAGNESIA: A COMPARISON

Comparison of remedies amounts to a differential diagnosis of therapeutic indications. As such it goes to the heart and core of the specific homeopathic approach. In comparing remedies, we actually compare constitutional responses and constitutional states of people.

Our basic premise for differential diagnosis is expressed in Hahnemann's formulation (Organon, Paragraph 7) that "since the totality of the symptoms is the outwardly reflected picture of the internal essence of the disease, it must be the principle or sole means whereby disease can make known what remedy it requires". This postulate represents an approach to therapeutics which insists upon dealing directly with perceived phenomena rather than with mental abstractions like our usual clinical concepts of disease syndromes, as useful as they may be for the purpose of theoretical classification.

A phenomenon (Greek: something that has become apparent, perceivable) is directly and immediately observable. An abstraction, in turn, is something that has been worked upon by thinking (often enough, tampered with by thinking) in the form of abstracting. To abstract (from the Latin abstrahere, to pull or draw away) is defined as mentally drawing away an isolated content from the connection or context in which it is originally found or perceived. This original context contains also other elements, the combination of which varies from case to case in an individual fashion. The abstraction, therefore, draws the common, that is, nonindividual, nondifferentiating elements out of the individual phenomena for the purpose of creating common denominators for remembering and classifying. Abstraction, therefore, by definition does away with the individual and individualizing qualities. It is concerned with quantities, statistical averages and common, nonindividual factors. No pneumonia that we ever encounter actually is the textbook pneumonia, which is an abstraction of the elements common to the greatest possible number of people with inflamed lungs. Every actually encountered case differs from this mental abstraction called pneumonia in his own individual fashion since no individual "is" the average. In turn, our modern clinical pathology deliberately and by definition limits itself to dealing only with such abstractions and with statistical averages. As a matter of principle this approach rejects the validity of the individual fact which is always a singular and unique one. Hahnemann based his whole approach upon the unique individual and individualized picture — the phenomenon rather than the abstraction. He follows in the footsteps of Paracelsus who (in vain) called upon the physician to hold on to nature itself rather than to speculation, since "nature is what can be seen but speculation (we used the word abstraction) is what cannot be seen. But it is the seeable rather than the unseeable that makes one a physician. The seeable renders the truth. The unseeable renders nothing. Everything that is invisible in us becomes visible. From this, it follows that you should not say this is cholera, that is melancholia but rather this is an arsenical that is an aluminous state." (Book Paragranum).

This quotation, by the way, shows us also Paracelsus' indications for his drugs seem quite in keeping with our modern experimental provings.

Thus, it is the differentiation of individual pictures, the arsenical, the aluminous that becomes the task of practical differential diagnosis rather than of disease concepts. The disease concept gives us merely an average of general prognosis and expectation (to be sure, is valuable too) but not a practical way of helping a given individual case.

The main colouring elements of these pictures are contributed by the general and mental symptoms. Furthermore, in comparing disease pictures with remedy pictures, symptom totality with symptom totality, we create not only fundamentally new constitutional classifications; actually entirely new concepts are introduced into physiology and pathology. Arsenic, Aluminum, Calcium, Magnesium are not merely substances. They are recognized as representing energy fields of specific physiological qualities. Their integration or disintegration within the "whole" of the organismic balance finds its concrete phenomenological expression in health or disease, nay *is* health or disease. We begin our medical study with the consideration of the curative agents and not of the causes of disease, since "it is the cure that shows us the cause of disease" says Paracelsus right at the beginning of his Volumen Paramirum. The likeness of the state that therapeutically responds to Calcium is the Calcium energy field in a state of one-sided preponderance which disbalances the whole. This statement is a simple verbalisation of empirically established phenomena. In the form of expressing those facts, we follow the method of modern physics which conceives of the universe not any more in terms of the mechanistic interaction of "things" but of dynamic interactions of energy fields — that is, force patterns — simply more modern words for the same entity that Hahnemann called "spirit like" force or dynamics. Thus our differentiation of remedies is a differentiation of qualitatively distinguished energy fields which are building stones of our peculiar human nature. What we have called drug pictures are pictures of people, of states of personality, of living and suffering. The perception of such pictures, in what otherwise would be a maze of disjointed facts, allows us to see a pervading oneness in an otherwise confusing multiplicity of symptoms. It provides us with a red thread of meaning around which we can arrange in a logical fashion those symptoms that otherwise would be an endless maze of irrelevant facts which have to be committed to memory in a mechanical fashion.

In this sense, we proceed to a specific instance of comparing the state of *Calcarea* with the state of *Magnesia,* the quality of the *Calcarea* energy field with the pattern of the *Magnesia* energy field.

The very act of comparing and differentiating two things implicity postulates their basic similarity. In the case of *Calcarea* and *Magnesia,* that basic similarity of constitutional action appears but insufficiently appreciated so far in our Materia Medica. Before differentiating the two drugs, some attention is due, therefore, to their common features first. This is the more important practically since a good many of the less known *Magnesium* indications (our *Magnesium* symptomatology being quite fragmentary) are simply duplications of *Calcarea* indications. The ignorance of this fact will make the prescriber consider *Calcarea* only, in the face of symptoms which would actually call for *Magnesium.*

Let us recall first that *Calcium* and *Magnesium* belong to the same group of the periodic system of elements; the so-called earth-alkalis include Calcium, Magnesium, Barium and Strontium. In the electrolyte balance of cells and tissue liquids, Calcium and Magnesium ions are synergistic and mutually exchangeable to a certain extent. With Sodium and Potassium, Calcium and Magnesium are the four principal cations of Ringer's solution, which duplicate the physiologic salt balance of the body fluids. Sodium and Potassium increase tissue irritability, Calcium and Magnesium reduce it. Sodium and Potassium do not pass readily through the cell membranes; their action is primarily in the tissue liquids. The earth-alkalis in turn are centered in their activity in the formed structural elements, the tissues themselves — particularly, muscles and bones. They affect the permeability of the cell membranes and (in the case of Calcium) the blood clotting. The earth-alkalis, thus, are functionally connected with formation, solidification and action of the tissues proper as they delimit themselves against the liquid medium out of which they are formed. They seem to be builders of solid ground in the organism just as in the mineral sphere of the earth, they precipitate and solidify the sedimentary rock formation out of the flowing waters. In most general terms, we may tentatively characterize the effect of Calcium and Magnesium as upon growth and structural organization as well as upon circulation.

Growth and structural organization include not only tissue (especially bone growth) but also the delimitation and maintenance of the body's own form principles against such exogenous or endogenous factors that would lead to disorganization. They encompass the organization of tissue liquids as well as the defense mechanisms against infective and allergenic elements as well as against endogenous — namely, nervous and endopsychic factors — that would upset the normal balance.

The protection of any functional organization against disturbances from outside, we may, in general, characterize as walling off. The protection against upsetting influences from within amounts to stabilization. Walling off and stabilization, thus, are most apt general descriptive terms to characterize broadly the energy pattern of *Calcarea* and *Magnesia.*

Clinically speaking, the constitutional expression of a disturbance in the sphere of walling off and stabilization is found in the symptoms which characterize that state that formerly was called scrophulosis or lymphatism; later, exudative diathesis, and today runs under the more fanciful name of allergic tendency. One author will ascribe it to a disbalance of the body chemistry. According to another, it is due to a disorder of the vegetative nervous system, or due to a hormonal imbalance, and a third one may describe it as a psychosomatic disorder. And indeed, all and any of these explanations seem to be correct and not mutually exclusive at all; if we but think in terms of formative energy patterns which include chemistry, hormones, nervous and psychological entities as individual means of qualitative manifestations. Thus, the broad functional concept of the morbus Calcarea or morbus Magnesia (to use Paracelsus' mode of expression) is an illness of disturbed protective organization and stabilizing equilibrium, exudative or allergic diathesis with all the possible ramifications of psychological, sympathic, parasympathic, serological, hormonal, biochemical nature that have been ascribed to it. It is the state which Hahnemann called Psora.

We find with *Calcarea and Magnesia* the tendency to disturbed assimilation and growth, poor nutrition and underweight; furthermore, asthma, hay fever, eczema, hives, the whole host of allergic conditions affecting skin and internal parts, the low general and skin resistance, the tendency to repeated colds, acute and chronic infections, pus formation, boils, abscesses, poorly healing and poorly functioning skin, enlarged inflamed and swollen tonsils and adenoids. Also common to both substances are a general rheumatic diathesis of both acute as well as chronic forms. Typical for their lymphatic state is also the pasty, pale or yellowish tinged colour of the generally unhealthy skin, a feature of both drugs.

In the sphere of the circulation, which is the main expression of what we may term the inner stabilizing balance, the disturbance expresses itself in states of violent congestions (affecting particularly the head region), ebullitions of heat, acutest fevers, excessive perspiration (worse head, worse at night) sensation of fullness with pulsating, constricting or bursting pains, clinical states of migraine and biliary colics. External vasoconstriction, internal vasodilation, internal congestion with cold, clammy skin and feeble, fast pulse, shock like states.

Into the circulatory disbalance, we may also classify the paradoxical modalities of lack of vital heat and aggravation from cold air and yet sensation of heat with a desire for cool drinks and cool air.

Chemically, the stabilizing, balancing function, in its failure, results in a shift of the hydrogen ion concentration to the acid side. Both *Calcium* and *Magnesium* are known as alkalizing buffer substances. A failure of this functional balance explains to us the symptom of "sourness" and acidity as heartburn stomach hyperacidity, sour diarrhea, sour sweats, sour smelling patients and the keynote of "sour babies".

Also fitting into the range of the stabilizing balancing function of both *Calcarea* and *Magnesia* is the tendency to spasmophilia, tetany, clonic constrictive states of heat, blood vessels, the biliary system and extremities in the sphere of their disturbance.

Mentally and on the personality level, the tendency of walling off and inner stabilization means a leaning towards separativeness and self-finding. While in its favorable aspect, this means independence; in its less favorable, one-sided exaggeration it is withdrawal from people, tendency to go it alone, loss of social contact, stubbornness and obstinacy, typical for both *Calcarea* and *Magnesia*.

Thus, for the common features. It is when we turn to the differentiating factors that the full individuality of each drug personality becomes apparent.

In our quest for something like a key to the meaning of the individualizing features of formative patterns, we look for phenomena in nature which seem most characteristically to express the prototype of the substance activity. In such an image, we may behold the force pattern that, like a guiding symbol, gives us an understanding of the manifoldness of the symptomatology. We find it for *Calcarea* in the formations of chalk and of the oyster shell; for *Magnesia* in the plant green, the chlorophyll and the characteristic lightning-like flash of the *Magnesium* explosion which even has been used for flash bulbs and formerly for incendiary bombs. The chlorophyll, the greenness of the plants, the very archetype of all greenness that is life and renewal, is that enzyme which aids in the synthesis of starch out of water and carbondioxide under the influence of light. We might say that through chlorophyll (the molecule of which is built around the *Magnesium* atom) light, water and air are condensed into matter; *Magnesium* helps to synthesize matter. In the *Magnesium* flash explosion, in turn, matter is destroyed, light and heat are generated. Here *Magnesium* represents destruction of matter. Between both of these poles — creation and destruction — moves the eternal restless flow of life which is activity in never ending restless evolution and change. "Birth and death, an eternal sea, a changing weaving, a glowing life" are the words Goethe puts into the mouth of the "Spirit of the Earth". True to

123

our image, we find a preponderance of *Magnesium* also in the seawater, the primordial source and origin of all primitive and undifferentiated life, never at rest in its flow of tides and up and down of waves.

In contrast, the symbol image of chalk and of oyster represent standstill, passivity and immobility, the antithesis to the restless flowing life activity.

Chalk consists of deposits of the remains of foraminifera, namely millions and millions of shells, remainders of tiny sea animals, sealife that has come to a standstill and has formed immobile rocks. The oyster shell, from which *Calcarea carb* is prepared, is the casing by which the flabby gelatinous oyster immobilizes itself and sticks to a rock. The oyster represents a form of animal life which has reduced activity to the barest minimum. Clinging to the rock, its only activity consists in opening and closing its shell. Thus, the calcification process represents standstill, immobilization, shell formation, walling off and firmness; in the human organism in addition to the skeleton, which to us symbolizes both firmness and stability of structure, as well death, calcification occurs where tissue dies, becomes necrotic and is taken out of the metabolic process. *Calcium* tightens the cell membranes, *Magnesium* increases permeability. *Calcium* is found as precipitate deposit in the bones; *Magnesium* mostly in ionized solution in the soft tissues that as activating elements envelop the passive bones, namely muscle and nerve tissue. Moreover, a particularly high amount of *Magnesium* is found in sperm, the very essence of active mobility.

While they are synergistic in respect to solidification, growth, balance and stabilization out of the liquid medium; *Calcium* and *Magnesium* are antagonistic to each other in their dynamic impulsation within that state which they have established. Bipartisan in foreign policy, as it were; they represent the tension between conservatism and radicalism within.

Magnesium represents motion, change, drive impulse, activity and direction, a centrifugal, invigorating, active, driving force; life that is borne out of creation and destruction, a positive outgoing influence.

Calcarea is standstill, passivity, immobility, clinging, restraining, peripherally enclosing, restricting, ingoing, negative on holding in receptive principle.

One is reminded of the tenet of Chinese philosophy which holds that everything in nature is based on the balance of what is called Yang and Yin forces. Yang is the principle that is masculine, hot, driving, active, outgoing in pulsating, symbolized by gold and the sun. Yin is feminine receptive, cool, moist, passive, quiet, immobile, symbolized by silver and by the earth. The old practice of acupuncture, which in Europe is meeting with increasing attention and acceptance again, is based on that concept of Yang and Yin. Also modern depth psychology has verified the soundness of that concept; also, psychic life can be understood in the light of the polar tension of opposites of Yang and Yin like qualities.

We may begin to comprehend the *Calcarea* state now when we view it as a stress or problematic situation of the level of the Yin forces; that is a stress situation that brings into one-sided preponderance or breakdown the forces of immobilization, defensive protection, separation, walling off and shielding off. Stagnation and standstill seems to prevail. With *Magnesium*, in turn, the picture is dominated by the stress or the problem arising from too much impulsation, activation and drive. Explosiveness, aggressiveness and spastic violence tend to prevail. Growth and stability, of course, depend on a balance of both sides, on impulsation and direction, as well as, on protection and organization; the *Calcium* and *Magnesium* field in its synergism represents the interplay of the centrifugally dynamic and the centripetally static forces.

We can see before our inner eye the oyster-like *Calcarea* type as the plump, passive, phlegmatic, indolent complacent person that the Materia Medica describes. Most of the problems stem from their passivity. They may be too open to influences from their surroundings, too easily affected, hypersensitive or too armored and isolated in order to compensate for their lack of ability to meet a challenge by initiative — thus, becoming stubborn and obstinate. Physiologically that same defenselessness and failure of adaptability and of meeting challenges, we find as hypersensitivity to rough weather, coldness, dampness and the lack of stamina and endurance.

They are devoid of initiative and courage, easily cowed, weepy, fearful, apprehensive and depressed; the compensating opposite appears as overexcitability with a tendency to spastic conditions.

In the less extreme expressions of the *Calcarea* type, we simply have a lack of endurance and of the ability to rebound. Also, muscular endurance and performance are reduced.

On the positive side of the ledger, those same qualities may make the *Calcarea* persons slow, conscientious workers who steadily plod along. They are reliable partners, the opposite of the erratic and unpredictable *Magnesium* type; they are satisfied to build patiently and drag stone upon stone in their work. Not too imaginative, they may do best when left alone and allowed to proceed independently. Thus, although often quite sociable, they may give the impression of obstinacy.

The further details of the *Calcarea* symptomatology which are known well enough, we may safely omit in this presentation after having brought out the basic characterizing features.

Rather let us concentrate on the less well-known *Magnesium.*

The *Magnesium* personality is characterized by activity out of bounds. It is in a state of continuous flash fires and explosions of endless emotional up and down of angry outbursts and fearful depressions. *Magnesium* may well be called the most violent, ill-tempered, erratic but also fearful and depressed remedy of our Materia Medica. Its nearest resemblance for comparison would be *Chamomilla*. But unlike the acute and transitory temper tantrum of *Chamomilla,* the *Magnesium* state is the expression of a permanent constitutional personality pattern.

We deal here with people of a basic central emotional imbalance and unsteadiness. They helplessly are under the sway of their drives and impulses. The patients are excessively oversensitive, hysterical, irritable and subject to the extremist forms of emotional tensions. They are utterly unable to control their emotions or impose any amount of self-discipline upon them; subject to violent rages, fury, temper tantrums, the terror of the family or of the office should they be in charge. Full of fears and anxieties, children screaming at the sight of the doctor. Here we may remember that often fear is the reaction to one's own repressed, unconscious violence. Hypochondriacs, who are sure that every trifling indisposition is a catastrophical illness without hope for recovery, eternal complainers, violent bosses, patients in a state of nervous exhaustion but also, in the writer's own experience, borderline near psychotic cases marked by fear or depression. It definitely would deserve a trial as a most promising drug in manic depressive, as well schizophrenic patients whenever the symptoms agree. (In the actual near psychotic states of my own experience, most frequently, the indication was for *Magnes. mur*).

Not infrequently, the mental state is marked by a seemingly quiet and composed disposition. In these cases, the stormy, touchy violence is either hidden under a mask as the family will tell you or a discipline imposed by strongest will-power has succeeded in driving the stormy emotions underground. Such people, if they are of the *Magnesium* constitution, may then suddenly find themselves on the verge of a nervous breakdown descending upon them out of the blue sky. Or the repressed violence, deprived of the emotional outlet, expresses itself in its physiologic equivalent in storms of the autonomic nervous system. Just as it is the most temperamentally imbalanced, so *Magnesium* is also the most violently spastic and neuralgic drug of our Materia Medica. (This is true of all *Magnesias,* not merely the phosphate).

The spasms affect the visceral muscles, for instance, bronchial asthma, intestinal biliary, renal colics, etc; they affect the blood vessels as retinal spasms (visual disturbances) dizzyness, migraine due to constriction of the arteries of the head region and coronary condition (*Mag. phos)*. Finally, we find spasms in the extremities with ischemia, coldness, paresthesia, anesthesia and even states of shocklike nature with external coldness, nausea and cold sweat. The neuralgias may affect any nerve group and are often of the paresthetic type.

Next and in closest interplay with the autonomic nervous system are the ductless glands. The mental state of explosive, restless drive is most closely reflected in a hyperactivity of the thyroid gland. And indeed, the reproving of *Magnesium* carried out by Metzger, Stuttgart, Germany, demonstrated a pronounced effect upon the thyroid but also upon the prostate gland. Next to *Iodium, Magnesium* is first and foremost to be considered as a remedy in states of hyperthyroidism, toxic goiter, as well as thyroid heart. The symptoms produced in the provings were: swelling, pressure sensation and tenderness, choking and sensitivity to clothes pressure in the thyroid and neck area; heart palpitations, tachycardia, stitching pains in the heart area.

With this tendency to toxic goiter, we see again a confirmation of the complementary relationship to *Calcarea* which produces and cures fibrous goiter. Also here, *Magnesium* represents the overactive driving versus the slowing and arresting tendency of *Calcarea.*

The second important organotropic relation is to the prostate gland, thus suggesting that this gland about whose function we know so little, may perhaps have something to do with the masculine aggressive drive. In the provings, the sex drive may be increased or decreased; there is pressure and stiching pain in prostate and testicles, worse after urination and defecation. In clinical prostate hypertrophy, where our medical armamentarium leaves still much to be desired, the *Magnesias* are among the leading most frequently indicated remedies.

Metzger draws attention to the fact that in the family ascendancy of *Magnesium* types, one frequently finds hyperthyroidism which ipso facto is a potential *Magnesium* indication. He therefore suggests there may be a familial incidence of the *Magnesium* constitution by dominant inheritance. Thus, when having one *Magnesium* case in a family, one may do well to consider possible *Magnesium* indications for any other member of that family who either does not respond to the apparently indicated remedy or fails to show clear prescribing symptoms or, most important, looks like a *Calcarea* case on the surface, yet fails to show sufficient progress under *Calcarea.*

Magnesium, like *Calcium,* has rheumatic diathesis. But whereas *Calcarea* primarily affects the joints, the *Magnesium* rheumatism, in line with general characterization, prefers the muscles and nerves with contractive, spastic and neuralgic states.

Another important *Magnesium* symptom is acyclical intermittency and changeability of symptoms. For no apparent reason, symptoms change, disappear and after a few weeks have elapsed, reappear again.

In their modalities, *Calcarea* and *Magnesia* differ inasmuch as *Mag-*

nesium is better from walking in the open air. *Magnesium* is aggravated by riding in a carriage (carsickness), from sweets and fat (particularly *Mag. sulf)*. Also, the *Magnesias* are among the "dizziest" remedies. Both are chilly and worse from coldness.

Both, the *Calcarea,* as well as the *Magnesia* states, are most typically represented in the symptomatology of the carbonates. Since our Materia Medica lists a fair amount of symptomatology as far as the particulars of *Mag. carb* and *Mag. mur.* are concerned, the further details may be studied there and need not be referred to here.

A few words may be in place, however, in respect to the differentiating features of the various *Magnesium* compounds.

Magnesia mur. seems characterized by a particularly marked depressive tendency. A dark gloom has settled which may be temporarily interrupted by explosions of violence. Since the picture reminds one of *Natrum mur.* (but is far in excess of the *Natrum mur.* depression), one may wonder whether there is not a certain accentuation of a depressive character inherent in the chloride ion. *Magnesia mur.* deserves attention in psychiatric conditions.

With the phosphate, we are also fairly familiar. Not sufficiently appreciated is the fact, however, that *Mag. phos.,* like all *Magnesias,* has a broad range of deep and long lasting constitutional effects. The *Magnesia phos.* type is, as we would expect from the foregoing, similar to the *Calcarea phos.* patient. They are the same thin, weak, and sensitive types, with the same nutritional, psoric and allergic problems, yet characterized by the fiery magnesium impulsivity rather than the calc. passivity. They often are thin, dark complexioned, very sensitive artistic or intellectual people, extremely nervous, intense, restless, spastic, and neurotic with cramps and colics all over; foremost, we mention angina pectoris, chorea paralysis agitans, but also professional neuroses like writer's cramp, etc., in addition to the other well-known indications.

Magnesium jodatum is dark, scrawny, shriveled, thin and worn out, is in a state of continuous uproar or depression. It combines the features of two of the most restless drugs we know of. Its special indications are hyperthyroidism, prostatic and biliary condition.

Mag. sulf. (Epsom salt) has a special affinity to liver, biliary, pancreatic and intestinal disturbances. I have been watching a case of prostate hypertrophy gradually improving over three years now with *mag. sulf.* Its special features are aggravation from fats, from riding trains, diarrhea with great thirst, diabetes with great thirst, and polyuria, disseminated warts of children, depression, fits of passion, beside themselves with forebodings and anxiety. The sulfur component is quite obvious.

In our differential diagnostic comparison, we have given more attention to *Magnesium* than to *Calcarea*. It is hoped that this comparative stress upon the less well-known of the two earth alkalies will help to restore to its deserved place in the scope of our prescribing, one of the most important drugs of our homeopathic armamentarium.

In thinking in holistic terms, Hahnemann was ahead of his as well as our time with his anticipation of an overall pattern which encompasses not only substance but also what we now call energy. This was his most revolutionary discovery, a oneness that underlies illness and cure as one and the same. Both have begun to be repostulated in our time by modern physics, biology and depth psychology.

We no longer hold what is called the billiard ball theory of matter, namely the pushing around of intert particles of matter by what is called energy. We now acknowledge that matter and energy are actually one, neither having an independent reality but dependent on each other on transitory manifestations of what is called 'form,' nothing but form. Process of form is the underlying unit of existence. This is not form of something, but form per se, prior to any 'thing'; form creating that which we call matter. This sounds like an abstruse notion, yet I would remind you that we change all the atoms and molecules of our body within approximately seven years, yet the person seems the same one. How do we recognize this sameness? By virtue of the determining form principle, the elements of form that create or precede our material existence.

Similarly, biology thinks in terms of what Portmann has called 'themes'—themes expressing themselves in the creation of forms. This idea overrides the Darwinistic idea of chance selection in terms of survival value. He describes for instance the descent of the testicles as having no survival value. Outside of the abdominal cavity the testicles are more exposed to danger than before and this location does not serve survival. Likewise many animal forms such as the shape of a horn or thickened skin folds in no way serve as life preserving or biological functions but rather express creative plays of existence. Nature is an artist creating and shaping forms for its own ends. As Goethe said: "The phenomena are their own explanation. They need no further explanation."

Similarly in depth psychology, particularly in terms of Jung's concepts, complex and archetype are seen as both the origin as well as the healer of a disorder depending upon whether these autonomous principles can be integrated into an overall wholeness in life and living or whether they operate independently as disturbing factors.

All of these concepts add up to the idea of form or Gestalt, elements that are more than the sum of their parts, the parts being integrated in an overall pattern by the law of the form. This is the angle that Hahnemann intuited in creating what he called the 'Arzneimittle Bilder,' namely the pictures or images of remedies as though they were personalities, *Miss Pulsatilla, Mr. Sulphur* or *Mrs. Sepia.*

You may say that in the realm of creative forms they do exist. This is what is meant with the genius of the remedy, namely an underlying core of meaning, a form significance that shapes something that we treat as if it were an image, a person or a part of a personality.

What I want to draw to your attention is that this is not a playful fantasy but a working hypothesis tested in clinical use by depth psychology. Our psychic system actually perceives and operates in terms of such form patterns. The form elements are world creating forces, entities, the power of God or whatever you want to call them.

Our remedy pictures then constitute what is called in German, 'Sinnbilder.' Translated, Sinnbild means image of meaning or symbol. Through the symbol we grasp the way the cosmic and biological energy forces operate meaningfully. The symbolic model is used now in nuclear physics, in depth psychology and to a certain extent in modern biology but has not as yet, by and large, reached the science of medicine. But it is unconsciously inherent in Hahnemann's approach. I now propose to use the symbolic approach for the sake of understanding more fully the dynamic force of the serpent, the snake remedies, foremost of which is *Lachesis.*

Let me digress for a moment and say that also a good deal of clinical pathology can be understood in terms of body symbolism. It is for instance true that when you analyze the psychosomatic background of cardiac disorder, you will nearly always find very central feeling problems that have been repressed. This is in keeping with old tradition, old intuitive insight of the heart symbolising the functions of feeling. In gastric or duodenal ulcers, you might think, 'What is eating this person emotionally?' This is an organism that devours itself. The typical rheumatic state somehow indicates a rigidity, a tendency to be found in the personality as well as the body.

Also in psychiatric understanding of the unconscious psyche we proceed by relating its dynamics of dream and phantasy images to mythological and symbolic motives (themes) which are the language of the unconscious psyche. Mythological symbolism offers most ancient as well as the most modern, hence timeless, comprehension of man's relationship with cosmic forces.

Now let us look at the image pattern, the Gestalt or form, the symbol of the serpent as though it were a dream of nature in which a particular state of man, a particular potential state of pathology is represented. The serpent is one of our most ancient and most grandiose mythological motives. I would remind you that the staff of Aesculapius features the serpent wound around a central staff. The

131

serpent is the image of primordial, autonomous, impersonal life energy underlying and creating existence and consciousness. It is the image of the instinctual life will, of desirousness, hunger for life, (Latin, libido), the urge to taste life, to learn and grow through tasting life. In Eastern tradition it represents what is called Maya, namely the illusion as well as reality of existence, the manifestation of primordial energy, Prakriti. You are given a feeling about the consciousness-offering quality of the snake in the Old Testament, its creative force is more masked in the popular version than in esoteric tradition. And lastly, Hahnemann referred to it when he prefaced his Organon "Aude Sapere: Dare to taste and understand." Sapere means both taste and understand. Hence the snake force involves us in life and living, not theoretically, merely, but by deeply emptying the cup. It is a force which is wrapped around the tree of life in the story of paradise which led to the fall from paradise but also to life's healing forces in the staff of Aesculapius.

You also find the serpent on the cross substituted for Christ in the Christian Gnostic tradition. It is that which involves the fall of man and again leads him out from it. The serpent is to be elevated, to be brought to a higher level. It is the force which leads to life and into life and is being developed into consciousness, but, and here is the great paradox, in this development of consciousness life has turned against itself.

Therefore the image of the snake which eats its own tail, the uroboros, is the symbol of the infinity of life. In the development toward consciousness, toward an ego, life of necessity turns against itself. Ego development rests upon at least partial repression of instinctual urges. If we are not willing to live like animals, we must take a stand against our spontaneous emotional and instinctual drives; and this is the split within the life forces of the serpent itself. It is a de-integration, a fragmentation which rends the harmonious wholeness. Where logos opposes bios, spirit stands against life and you encounter the pathology of the serpent. The serpent pathology is the unintegrated life impulse, the unintegrated libido, the unintegrated instinct split off and split in itself. It is the rebellion or paralysis of the life urge or libido; you can say *Lachesis* is the penalty of unlived life. Thus you have the egocentricity of *Lachesis* and on the other hand, the motif that appeared in the dream in Dr. Stubler's paper of which the depth psychological symbolism is quite evident. The motif of cutting up one's own husband means cutting one's own unconscious maleness. Cutting up the 'totally other,' namely the unconscious side, amounts to the destruction of the unconscious libido. Let me say in parenthesis that the rubric on dreams in Kent ought to be taken with a grain or several grains of salt. They often fit but owing to the lack of psycho-dynamic understanding of dream symbolism one can easily be led

132

astray. This is a dream which I would say is indeed typical of *Lachesis* inasmuch as the woman is severing herself psychologically from all the life impulses, but it need not refer only to *Lachesis.*

The main heading of serpent pathology is the repression and cutting off of vital forces as a price to be paid for personal and personality development. This covers all that which Hahnemann intuited under the heading of Psora, the universal sickness of man. Consequently Kent's remark that the basic snake nature is what we all have. In a way, I would consider the snake venom a most acute anti-psoric medicine.

Now, I would say *Lachesis* is a particular, special version of this, as all snakes have their own personalities and diversions of pathology. *Lachesis* represents what I would call a jungle variety of this libido aspect. It is the emotionally and sexually charged picture which reminds me somewhat of a chronic Gelsemium with its sultry sensuousness. It is something like a thick smell of repressed emotionality and sensuality which makes me think of *Lachesis.*

Now, having this model in view, how does it establish a sense of order among the chaos of clinical and proving symptoms? How does it apply to the *Materia Medica?* Let us take the guiding symptoms one by one. First: the left sidedness or left to right; here you have an extension, an invasion as it were, of pathology from the left side. The left side is the sinistra side, the sinister side because left has always been equated with the unconscious functioning. It is the heart side, the relatively receptive, not to say passive side. Therefore it is the feeling and emotional side. You will find that the left side is always overburdened emotionally and programmed toward the unconscious; with all this we also think of Sepia and Phosphorous. Also these are predominantly unconscious-determined, oversensitive, even clairvoyant medicines. *Lachesis* also has this as well as *Sepia,* a heavily repressed emotional type. You have here the classical, typical invasion of repressed energy from the unconscious, emotional personality.

The next keynote is constrictiveness, constriction anywhere but particularly of the throat. I find this as a psychiatric syndrome quite frequently when the capacity to ascertain oneself as a personality is threatened. The globus hystericus for instance is a typical response for the throat when the ego has a difficult time holding its own against the invasion of emotional and especially sexual forces. The constrictiveness is a response to unseen yet powerfully experienced forces.

Next is the breakdown of the blood life and the autonomous nerve control. You may remember that the Nazi slogan was "Blood and Soil." With all its viciousness in the political circumstances this was a psychologically profoundly moving symbolic image. It would not have been so vicious, had it not been so valid. Blood is indeed the deepest, most basic expression of life and living. When life is repressed, the regeneration of the blood-element is disturbed. The constriction of blood, of life force constricts physiologically in analogy to the psychological image of cut off emotion. Think of the anemic Victorian young ladies whose goodness did not allow them to live a red blooded life.

Finally, the epitome of unlived life is to be found in the tendency for carcinoma. To me cancer is number one on the list of psychosomatic disorders arising from unlived life which concretizes as autonomously unintegrated growth which then exceeds the total organism and does not fit into the whole. In cancer pathology you will always find a sense of hopelessness, disappointment, bitterness, grimness, resentment against existence, whether events precipitate these feelings or not. Even in the Rohrschach pattern these personality traits have been confirmed, namely the constrictive, overcontrolled personality that has come to the point of breakdown of these controls. It is not merely the 'repressed' personality, since everyone nowadays is found to be repressed in one way or another but specifically the personality repressed with respect to the life supporting qualities of aggression, emotion and sexuality. It is a repression of the emotional intensity: violent intensity underlying a controlled surface. Hence this personality is suspicious to the degree of paranoia, tense and depressed. I do not believe too much in the vaunted jealousy as a leading or helpful symptom because, as in the case of repression, everyone has it. Rather the condition is similar to that of a snake lying quiescent ready at the slightest provocation to strike, to bite. With a susceptibility to hallucinatory and ecstatic states the slightest cause triggers the crack that may lead to explosion.

From this standpoint the intense aggressive urge is also more comprehensible. The *Lachesis* personality is so uptight and the underlying tendency to close off hides a vicious hate, meanness and even cruelty: the revenge for a life not lived. There is restraint, a seeming shyness overlaying a bitter tongue. We also find states that are the result of grief, fright, suppressed love, encountered danger or sorrow which could not be integrated into the overall feeling life of the personality. The life flow is stopped, blocked on both the physical as well as the psychological level. Body juices, menstrual or other are blocked in their flow. So it is understandable that a keynote of *Lachesis* is improvement from the opening of discharges.

Lastly the climactic point, the last chance at the change of life for the juices to flow. The change of life represents a critical point for the *Lachesis* symptomology. In this last chance situation the life force and the emotions produce something akin to the eruption of a volcano.

There is also aggravation from sleep. In sleep all of our conscious controls are relaxed. The same, by the way, applies to the effects of alcohol, also a keynote of aggravation. The consciously controlled

134

activities are relaxed and the unconscious can take over, and it takes its compensating revenge. When we wake up, what do we find? We find ourselves overwhelmed by all the forces and impulses we cannot consciously accept and permit. We try to pull down the lid again, and conflict and aggravation ensue from the rebound toward repression.

Aggravation from touch. You know when you are pressed or hit, psychologically, you bound back, but when the soft approach is used, you are 'touched.' Your feeling overrules your defenses and comes forth. This is what the *Lachesis* person's repressed life feelings and emotions cannot afford. Touch evokes the feeling, evokes the emotion and thus evokes the aggravation of the repressed tendencies. But on the other hand, hard pressure improves because we can respond with a tightening and shaping up to the pressure. However, there is an over-sensitivity to anything constricting, because the constrictive tendency is a threat to vital functioning. This is a poignant example of how body functioning taken symbolically reflects the working of the archetype.

Finally we have aggravation in the autumn but foremost in the spring. These seasons of transition, of budding love and life lower the conscious defenses and are times of *Lachesis* aggravation. Conversely, motion, cold, fresh air, wakeful activity stimulate conscious control and close the lid effectively on the intense unconscious upsurge.

Let us now consider the development of organ pathology, head, throat, heart, ovary and veins, and blood decomposition.

The head is the center of ego consciousness. When pathology is no longer held in check, the superiormost controlled organ breaks down first. When a revolt succeeds, it topples the ruling chiefs first. Take for instance migraine headaches: migraine expressing the psychological state of forcing one's head through a wall. The wall doesn't suffer but the head does.

The throat area we have already characterized as the area of conflict between continued control of the sense of identity on the one hand and the onrush of unconscious emotions on the other.

The heart is the center and the seat of the validating of life qualities and life feelings.

The ovaries and sexual organs evidently are the center of repressed libido, sexual and biological urges.

The veins are the channels where the life flow becomes relatively turgid. Remember again the image of the sultry jungle world of *Lachesis*. As the life flow slows, stagnation sets in in waters already stilled. Whatever the organ, whenever the lower half of the body is reached by the repressive effects, the vital functions are most centrally threatened.

I have attempted to give you a sense of the personality traits of *Lachesis*, the Gestalt underlying isolated keynote symptoms that you may recognize this picture of repressed intense life urge pushing back in the pathological state of *Lachesis*.

I believe that the readiness to perceive these holistic, psychosomatic, indeed personality patterns which is now, albeit slowly, making its advent into some branches of modern psychology may be able to bring us a step nearer to the profound mystery of Homeopathy.

The mystery of Homeopathy is close to the mystery of life; it is the paradox of the hidden unity of suffering and healing, the very mystery of the serpent wound around the tree of life: the emblems of Hermes the guide of souls and of Asclepius the Healer.

CARBO ANIMALIS

The carbons are the main building stones of living matter. All organic chemistry is based and structured on the carbon molecule. *Carbo Animalis* and *Carbo Veg.* are precipitates of living and dying organisms. They are stages of incomplete combustion, oxidation not carried to the ultimate product of carbon dioxide but prematurely precipitated. They represent incomplete life cycles. The converting of living organic substance into combustion products is a basic life process: through 'living breath', through oxidation we convert living matter into carbon dioxide. The appearance of incompletely oxidized carbons would indicate an incomplete or unsatisfactorily completed life process, the inability to complete the process. The full consummation, oxidation of the life process occurs with age and is completed in death. Here one might compare the inadequate living of one's potential, of consummating emotional tensions, griefs, joys and working through paradoxes and conflict to the incomplete combustion of carbon.

We meet the pathology of the aging process, regardless of actual age, in *Carbo Animalis* and *Vegetablis*. The *Carbo veg.* patient may be likened to a state of vegetative disturbance and breakdown: the limitations of a gradually declining vitality, a slower metabolism, resulting in imbalance of combustion of unconverted waste. On the *Carbo animalis* level we meet the "animalic," the imbalance of oxidation. Repressed and unconsummated emotional functions exert pressure and interfere with physiological balance.

Thus the pathology of *Carbo animalis* could be understood as the difficulty of acceding to the demands of aging and maturing on the instinct and affect level. When receptivity, tolerance and the inability to change come to a halt the result is isolation, rigidity and anxiety.

The Materia Medica describes a state of isolation, rejection of people, withdrawal and withering. These people become slaves to their own rigid views and routine; they respond with anxiety to the threat of any disturbance of their accustomed way of thinking or living. The result is a gradual failure of adaptibility per se. One interesting detail is the symptom of confused hearing, of confusion and failure to locate the direction from which sounds come. Adequate hearing reflects the capacity of receptivity. In hearing we take in from the outside. If this function is disturbed, we lack orientation to the outside, to our fellow beings.

The personality type may be described as introverted, indrawn, scrawny, thin, dark, sometimes heavy set, rigid, retiring, antisocial with an aversion to people, desiring to be alone. The *Carbo animalis* patients are poor mixers, though they may enjoy the company of one or two individuals to whom they are accustomed. Newcomers are not admitted. Throughout the symptomatology runs aversion and incapacity to deal with change. The symptom of homesickness is actually the state of not being content away from the accustomed known, rather than any expression of human attachment. There is aversion to conversation, taciturnity, shyness, a feeling of isolation, often heard in the words, "When I was young..."; a mournful reflective state of discouragement and gloominess, obstinate irascibility, ill humor, a feeling of being abandoned, thoughts of death and hopelessness.

The reaction of the psyche to this state of repressive isolation is anxiety, fear of the dark, fear in the evening, fear when going to sleep; fear breaking in whenever ego control weakens. Then the repress-level rises. The same incapacity to adapt expresses itself on the physical level also. The slightest change of routine is intolerable. Weakness, exhaustion and aggravation result. The patient finds it difficult to get started and resents being prodded or hurried. The slightest disturbance in physical health is aggravating. There is a lack of adaptation also in the digestive system expressed in frequent intestinal upsets. Almost anything may upset the digestion. Even normally harmless food will present problems which the weak assimilative power of the organism cannot handle.

The general constitutional state expresses a tendency to 'stay put', to stagnate, harden. Foremost is the cancerous hardening. This is the area for which *Carbo animalis* has been used routinely, unfortunately so, in view of the much wider range of pathology which belongs to its scope. If there were a simple description of cancer, of the constitutional or psychological aspect of cancer, it could be characterised as 'life inadequately lived', of hardening prematurely and onesidedly. Cancerous hardening, hardening glands, hard scirrhous growths are leading keynotes but we have equally hardening of joints and muscles, chronic rheumatism in any and every form. These rheumatic symptoms have not been given adequate evaluation in our prescribing. We have arthritic stiffness, gouty nodosities, tension in the limbs as if tendons were contracted, numbness and spasmodic contractions all over. The psychosomatic aspect of rheumatism is one of defensive rejection, of stiffening against aggressiveness and emotion.

The weak joints, easily sprained, point again to the failure of adaptive strength and flexibility. So do the venous congestions, ebullitions of heat (circulatory lack of adaptation) and the already mentioned lack of digestive adaptation.

Among the modalities the general air hunger characteristic for both carbons may express inadequate oxidation, inadequate cellular respiration or combustion. We find aggravation from cold and dry air, reflecting the lack of adaptility of the circulatory, capillary system and of warmth regulation.

In the psychopathology of obesity which occurs to a certain extent in *Carbo animalis,* there is a tendency to compensate for emotional starvation with sweet, fat and starchy foods. The problem is that the *Carbo animalis* patient also lacks the capacity to assimilate these foods.

POLYCHREST VERSUS LESS FREQUENTLY USED REMEDY — ADDITIONAL SYMPTOMS OF LACTRODECTUS MACTANS

As a rule, a case defies our efforts to find the curative remedy not because there is no remedy which would cover its symptom totality, but because we have failed to consider or to recognize this remedy. Every single substance of the mineral, plant and animal world represents a potential medicine which may be required in a given disorder. Of all these millions of therapeutic possibilities even the most encompassing of all, Boericke's *Materia Medica,* lists only approximately twelve hundred. Of the majority of these we have only a fragmentary knowledge of symptoms for exact prescribing to perhaps a hundred of the best proven polychrests.

It is often held that a thorough knowledge of those polychrests is sufficient to cover every case with which we may be confronted. After all, these drugs are polychrests because their nature and composition bear such a fundamental relation to the human organization that the majority of disorders requires their prescription. On the other hand we ought to admit to ourselves that, because we are more familiar with them than with the other medicines, we tend to lean upon the polychrests more heavily than is sometimes justified by the patients' needs. No remedy can ever take the place of the simillimum. Undoubtedly, the polychrests are the most basic substances and of deep action. Yet, when a remedy of only a superficial sphere of action happens to be indicated by the symptoms, any other one, though of constitutionally deeper repute, will act no better than distilled water. Often we meet with reference to certain drugs as "good" or "bad" remedies for this or that. This way of thinking is contrary to the basic idea of Homeopathy. There are no "good" or "bad" medicines, only indicated or not indicated medicines. *Sulphur* or *Calcarea* may be quite "bad" medicines and some little obscure herb with but a supposedly superficial effect a "good" one, if required by the symptoms of the individual case.

It has been the writer's experience that from among every ten patients, seven or eight on the average will actually require and satisfactorily respond to a polychrest. The remaining two or three, however, require a more unusual remedy, at least temporarily. From among these cases we recruit the bulk of our failures and unsatisfactory improvements. Often we assume obstacles to recovery where the only obstacle lies in our yet fragmentary knowledge of the *Materia Medica.*

The case presented in this paper at first defied the best efforts of diagnosis and prescribing. Failing to respond to the apparently well-indicated polychrests, this case furnished valuable, well-defined symptom material for the relatively unproven drug which turned out to be the correct simillimum.

Mrs. S., 36 years old. Two years before the onset of the present illness she had lost a little son through an accident. She never regained her peace of mind. During the preceding months she was under great additional strain, emotionally and physically, caring for her disabled parents. At the end of December, 1948, in a state of utter physical and emotional exhaustion, she contracted a cold. A few days later, on the exact anniversary of the child's death, she was completely immobilized by an excruciating pain in the right lumbosacral area. The next day found her unable to void urine and to move her legs. Examination showed an area of muscular constriction along the lower spine with somewhat accentuated but normal reflexes and undisturbed skin sensorium.

However, the patient was in a state of frenzied restlessness, screaming and crying with pain, unable to lie still, yet aggravated by any motion. There was no urge for stool whatsoever and urination could be induced only by pouring warm water over the perineum. The temperature was between 99.5 and 100°. An orthopedic specialist ruled out a slipped or ruptured disc, though an incipient caries remained a remote possibility. The modalities were: worse at night; very chilly, yet better open air; tearful disposition; restlessness; and the fact that the last period had been extremely scanty, almost completely suppressed. Rx: *Pulsatilla* 200. Relief moderate and short-lived. *Pulsatilla* 1M followed by a temperature rise to 101°. For a day the pains became somewhat more tolerable. The paralysis, on the other hand, increased. The possibility of a myelitis was considered now, and neurological consultation was requested. The neurologist, one of the best men in his field, at first leaned toward the diagnosis of a myelitis; then, learning about the emotional background was more inclined to consider it a conversion hysteria. Since the family was extremely alarmed, he suggested immediate hospitalization for a diagnostic "work-up." Before she was taken to the hospital the symptoms were reviewed again. Additional features now were an extreme drum-like distension of the abdomen, loud belching, nausea, loss of appetite, at times brownish vomiting, a great thirst for cold water which was taken in little sips, an aversion to sweets, an offensive odor from the mouth, and a feeling of heaviness and oppression on the chest. Still tearful with indefinite fears. The pain now cramping and shooting like waves of labor pains. *Phosphorous* 200. Upon arriving at the hospital the next day the pain was somewhat easier and the bladder function gradually became normal but the inactivity of the rectum remained. The patient remained in the hospital for about five weeks with all diagnostic and therapeutic attempts unavailing. She returned home unimproved and without definite diagnosis. However, the homeopathic study of the case could be resumed again. Now a status of utter exhaustion seemed to dominate the picture; in view of *Phosphorous* having done relatively the best, though failing upon repetition in the same as well as in a higher potency, *Phosphoric acid* 200, and later 1M was given. For several weeks the patient improved and became able to rise from her bed and move about, slowly and with support. However, the pains were still almost unbearable, particularly during the night, after the first sleep, and with every change of weather towards rain or electric storms. Mentally also, she was not better. After a few weeks *Phosphoric acid* did not elicit any further response. Additional symptoms now were flushes of heat and an inability to concentrate on any thoughts. *Lachesis, Sepia, Magnesia carbonica,* and *Rhus toxicodendron* gave absolutely no response.

Two months after the first onset of her illness, *Lactrodectus mactans* 200 was given. There was such an immediate and gratifying relief of all mental and physical symptoms that there can be no doubt that *Lactrodectus* was indicated from the very beginning. Within a few days the patient moved and walked freely and had only slight distress at night. Within two weeks she became practically normal.

Four weeks after this a sore throat occurred with desire for, and better from, cold drinks. *Mercurius solubilis* 200. given with little improvement; 1M improved the throat but brought back the backache with the patient generally worse. *Lactrodectus* 200. again removed the whole of the disturbance including the throat. Four and one half months after the onset, heart palpitations; hot flashes and chilliness; back pain on bending; sore throat and clogged up nose; soft, bleeding, spongy gums; ravenous appetite; and thirst again responded to *Lactrodectus* 200.

Subsequently, the toxicology of *Lactrodectus mactans,* the black widow spider, was studied. It was rather embarrassing to find that even the crude toxicological symptoms, as far as they are know, represent a perfect replica of this patient's condition. From the very beginning, even from the toxicological picture, the remedy would have been indicated had this picture only been known then to the prescriber. Unfortunately, however, *Lactrodectus* had been mentally associated with angina pectoris and nothing else, a very unhomeopathic attitude indeed.

The symptoms observed in clinical cases of spider bite, which were also outstanding in this case and removed by the potentized drug, should be added to our symptomatology of *Lactrodectus,* thus enlarging the scope of its use.

The following is a digest of this material which so far does not appear in any of our *Materia Medicas,* to my knowledge.

LACTRODECTUS MACTANS

The leading and determining features are:

Extremes of tension, spasticity, constrictiveness, and prostration.

They manifest themselves in the mind, the chest, the abdomen, the lumbar spine and the lower extremities in the first place.

The modalities are worst during the night; worse during damp weather and change of weather; worse before a thunderstorm; restless, tossing about but worse from motion and exhausted from every effort; chilliness; lack of vital heat but flashes of heat. Syphilitics and alcoholics are hypersensitive to *Lactrodectus;* alcohol especially aggravates all of its symptoms, thus suggesting alcoholism and constitutional syphilis among the general indications for *Lactrodectus.*

Mind: extreme restlessness; constant tossing around; fear; depression; hysteria; unrestrained and causeless crying in usually emotionally stable strong men.

General: extreme prostration; every effort is too much. Perhaps ill effects of overwork, etc. Muscle spasms with twitching, knotting, tremor, hyperactive reflexes and excruciating cramplike, unbearable pains, coming and going in waves like labor pains. Muscles sore to the touch. Worse motion, yet patient so restless that he cannot lie still.

Chest: angina pectoris; constrictive pain spreading to left shoulder and back; feeling of oppression; laboured respiration with an uncontrollable expiratory grunt. Palpitations of heart.

Abdomen: rigid as a board (defense musculaire?); distended like a drum. The distension is only slightly relieved by passing flatus. The whole picture most closely simulates an acute surgical emergency like perforated gastric ulcer, ruptured appendix and incipient peritonitis. (The temperature is subfebrile in the poisonings.)

Spine and back: the lumbar area shows the greatest degree of constriction; shooting, cramping pains; feeling as if the back were broken. Feeling of icy coldness from the hips downward. Paralysis of all functions associated with lumbosacral nerve plexus (genitals, urinary, rectum, lower extremities).

Extremities: paralysis; increased reflexes; spasticity; inability to lift legs because of spasm of the extensor muscles of the hips. Tenderness of the calf muscles upon palpitation; tingling sensation and numbness in hands and feet. Burning and stinging of the soles of the feet as if they were on fire. Swelling of ankles.

Head: headache (worse lying, better sitting?) probably congestive; tendency to apoplexy. Stuffiness of the nose.

Digestive: dry mouth, sore throat, great thirst for cold water which betters the throat, continuously drinking. Either loss of appetite or ravenous hunger. Vomiting of bitter brown matter. Extreme gaseous distension. Absolute inactivity of the rectum.

Female: menses suppressed, scanty, delayed.

Urinary: retention of urine; paralysis of the bladder; better warm application and pouring warm water over perineum.

Circulatory: flushes of heat followed by chilliness; apoplectic tendency, elevation of blood pressure; heavy perspiration. Temperature subfebrile.

The restlessness and constriction is shared with *Tarentula:* the coldness, worse from dampness, worse night and the neuralgic tendency with Aranea. However, Aranea has diarrhea and profuse menses; *Lactrodectus* has suppressed menstruation and constipation.

Lactrodectus presents itself as a medicine with characteristic symptoms of broad range and deep effect upon the vital force. It probably deserves an important place in our therapeutic armamentarium. We should consider it in acute emergencies of surgical as well as of circulatory nature, as well as in the spastic paralytic and neuralgic syndromes which conform with the mental and general symptoms thus far elicited.

REFERENCES

Blair, A.W., Spider Poisoning, Arch. Int. Med., 54:831, December, 1934.

Peple, W.L., Arachnidism: Report of a Case Simulating Diffuse Peritonitis. Virginia Medical Monthly, 56:789, March, 1930.

Thorp, R.W. and W.D. Woodson, Black Widow: America's Most Poisonous Spider, Chapel Hill: University of North Carolina Press, 1945.

Frank, L., The Black Widow Spider Bite Syndrome. Mil. Surgeon, 91:329, September, 1942.

Billmen, D.E., Arachnidism: With Report of a Case, U.S. Naval Medical Bulletin, 47:975, November-December, 1947.

Boericke, William, Homeopathic Materia Medica, 9th Edition. New York: Boericke and Runyon.

MANDRAGORA

Mandragora belongs among the oldest and most famous drugs used in ancient medicine as well as in magic. The more regrettable is it that for such a long time Homeopathy has failed to incorporate it into its exact armamentarium. Pythagoras called it humanlike because of its peculiarly shaped root which supposedly resembles a human body. Its medicinal use in antiquity was as an aphrodisiac (compare *Genesis* 30:14) as well as a hypnotic and analgesic. It was called *"morion"*, that is, the "root of madness" or of confusedness of the soul, the herb of Circe, the witch, who transforms men into animals through her love-magic. The mandrake was also considered the herb of Hecate, the dangerous goddess of magic, the mistress of the underworld and of demons, "Hecate chasing whining dogs, while walking across the graves of the dead and through dark streams of blood." (Theokritos). During the middle ages the "alraun," as it was then called, was considered a magical talisman that would bring luck and worldly goods; it was likened to a human body without a head, owing to the peculiar man-shape of the root. Thus, the symbolism makes it represent the forces of the body, the instinctual animalic "drives of the blood," as opposed to the spirit. Devoid of a head, it was supposed to receive a head through Christ, thus representing unredeemed mankind in need of salvation through divine grace. The Arabs called it "lamp of the devil." It was said to induce a revulsive nausea "like the smell of an adder."

Thus, we find that the "meaning" assigned to the mandrake, as expressed in this symbolic imagery arising from the collective unconscious of mankind throughout the ages, represents it as an entity of magic, animalic instinctuality, which is inimical to consciousness, confuses, intoxicates and arouses the force of the blood, the passions. The force of the herb puts a "magic spell" on man.

Now, in order to link such a concept with a practical symptom picture, let us imagine a person, who is under such a magic spell, exposed to the experience of a vision of Hecate, the "Black One," "the mistress over the evil demons who sends heavy sleep and oppressive dreams to man, who strikes with madness of love and passion"; of her who has been called the

> ...goddess of the crossroad, the glowing torch of the night, the enemy of light and friend of darkness who loves the baying of dogs and the spilling of blood, who walks over corpses, through dark streams of blood, over the graves of the dead, thirsting for blood and a horror to mortal man..."
> (— Hippolytos; Elenchos.)

Imagine anyone in the grip, under the power, of such a force. He is in a state of restless anxiety, confused, haunted, delirious; his vision becomes darkened, a prickling numbness is felt all over, every muscle and fiber gets tense, the blood rises to his head, a dizzyness overtakes him. His entrails, heart, stomach, bowels are contracted by fear and disgust, with nausea, vomiting or diarrhea and cramping or sticking pains resulting. His sexual instincts are aroused while yet his limbs stiffen in terror.

In this "phantasy image" we actually have given a description of the basic symptomatology of *Mandragora:* Drowsy hypnotic anxiety; numbness; darkening; of the vision; congestive states, particularly of head and abdominal and pelvic organs; extreme nausea; spastic states all over but foremost affecting heart, circulation and gastrointestinal tract; rheumatic stiffening of limbs.

The *Mandragora* pattern represents a condition of intoxication-like confusion and drowsiness with orgasms of blood, a state of quasi deadlocked excitation dissociated from purposeful body regulations.

Sleepiness, drowsiness, spasticity, numbness and *nausea* are the keynotes of the *Mandragora* picture, both psychologically and physiologically, in the mentals as well as the physical symptoms.

The *mental state* is characterized by a peculiar paradox of sleepiness and drowsiness with simultaneous intense excitement or excitability. We may call it apathetic irritability. The patients cannot sleep at night and are sleepy, yet overtense in the daytime. This is often typical for states of emotional frustration or instinct repression. Confused delirious states, overexcitability, oversensitivity particularly to noise, feelings of vague insecurity and anxiety, poor mental concentration, inertia, aversion to work, mental exhaustion and loss of memory. Changing moods, depression, crying spells alternating with euphoria and increased vital and mental activity or driving restlessness. They are oversensitive, "nervy" types, of hysterical or neurasthenic habitus, tending to hypomanic or actual manic-depressive states, often with vague ill-defined psychosomatic illness.

A typical *Mandragora* keynote is the occurrence of the mentals in association with nausea and numbness; for instance, inertia with nausea, depression or crying fits with nausea or numbness and relieved by profuse urination. (This relief by profuse urination is often the expression of a profound spastic repression in the emotional and sexual sphere.)

The *Mandragora* patient is always neurasthenic, hysterical or in a state of intensified emotional conflict with tension.

The sleep is restless and is often interrupted after midnight, especially 3 — 5 A.M., which is the general time of aggravation for *Mandragora.* I

146

have seen it relieve a delirious state characterized by loquaciousness, senseless irrational talking, blurred speech, with the patient knowing all the time what she wanted to say (the state is similar to that produced by the influence of liquor); inability to sit still, yet unable to walk, with a feeling as though the limbs were numb and paralysed. While this tallies with a state of being bewitched, this case, however, was due to a profound secondary anemia with a hemoglobin of about 20%. *Mandragora* 200. established a symptomatic normalcy and kept the patient going until she could be hospitalized for a blood transfusion.

Among the *general symptoms* anesthesia and hyperesthesia, numbness and dizziness stand foremost. Sensations of anesthesia or numbness in any part of the body, of whole nerve areas or in spots, sensation as though bugs were crawling over the whole body, loss of the sensation of touch, anesthesia of the mouth and the gums with petechiae and stomatitis; hyperesthesia, hypersensitivity to touch (but feeling better from deep pressure); uncontrolled spastic motions of the limbs.

Mandragora belongs among the dizziest drugs of our Materia Medica (alongside *Phosphorus, Conium, Magnesium*). It has faintness and fainting spells; the vertigo is often typical of Meniere's syndrome and comes in sudden attacks which force the patient to lie down; frequently, however, the dizziness is worse lying down, worse turning over, worse from motion and walking downstairs and worse upon awakening. Better from open air. Most frequently the vertigo is of emotional origin with an expressed feeling of insecurity, supposedly because of the dizziness; ill effects of anxiety and tension, dizziness with depression, or crying spells, ringing in the ears, or diarrhea.

The main organic structures affected by *Mandragora* are stomach, duodenum and liver-gallbladder area (tension, spasticity, gastritis, stomach and duodenal ulcers, cholecystitis, cholelithiasis); the circulatory system (hypertension, agina pectoris, coronary occlusion, gastrocardial symptom complex, functional circulatory disorders) and the locomotor system (neuritis, arthritis) as well as, in my own experience, congestion and inflammation in the areas of the head (2 cases of acute iritis).

Consequently lying, rest and relaxation, warm applications, passing secretions (urine, stool or eructations) improve. Bending over backwards often improves the abdominal colic and particularly the sciatica (cf. *Dioscorea*). The rheumatic pains are also better from continued motion. Damp weather, heat to the head and general coldness aggravate, since they increase stasis. Light touch aggravates, strong pressure improves. Eating improves the stomach symptoms.

HEAD: Congestive states. Sensation of fullness and heat; sensation as if head were shrinking. Pressure on top of head. Congestive headaches, better from cold air and cold applications. Head feels as in a fog. Worse from exposure to the sun, from alcohol, tobacco. Worse from touch, better from pressure. Headaches with diarrhea; headaches from anxiety, anticipation, etc.

EYES: Darkening of the visual field; all objects appear striped. Acute congestion of eyes. Styes, conjunctivitis, iritis.

EARS: Oversensitivity of hearing. Noises in the ears.

FACE: Facial herpes (cf. *Natr. mur.)*

HEART AND CIRCULATION: Palpitation of heart. Pains in heart, sticking or as though an iron ring would compress the heart. Numbness, choking sensation extending into left arm or to left shoulder with anxiety and a feeling of oppression. Worse at night, upon waking from sleep, motion and exertion. Better from rest, lying and warmth. Heart symptoms attended by intestinal symptoms, meteorism, distension, better from diarrhea. Gastrocardial symptom complex. Angina pectoris. Coronary infarction with states of shock and collapse.

Circulatory congestions, flashes of heat. Hot head, cold feet. Spastic constriction of the peripheral vessels (Reynaud's disease?) Hypertension.

MOUTH: Herpes labialis (cf. *Natrum mur.):* dryness; numbness; burning sensation as if burned with pepper; salivation; hemorrhagic stomatitis; stomatitis aphthosa; numbness in mouth.

THROAT: Tonsillitis.

STOMACH, ABDOMEN: Fullness; pressure in stomach; distension; eructations even with empty stomach, better from eating. Worse right side, better from passing gas. Worse after eating (immediately, or 1 − 2 hrs. later). Fullness and aversion to food upon beginning to eat. Hunger with aversion to food. Hunger pains, better from eating. *Pains better from bending backwards.* Intense nausea. Aversion to and worse from fats, coffee; desire for strongly tasting interesting foods (cf. *Puls.),* worse from sweets. Colicky pains with distension. Diarrhea or hard, small ball-shaped stools. Light colored stools. Tenesmus after evacuation, feeling as though not finished. Abdominal colic after midnight (12 − 2 A.M.). Pains in right upper abdomen radiating to right shoulder.

Hemorrhoids with burning sensation.

URINARY: Disturbed motor impulses. Frequent urge to urinate; dribbling of urine; urination difficult; urination involuntary.

Sexual libido increased or decreased (historical use as aphrodisiac). Menstrual cramps; menses intermittent. Uterine congestion, menorrhagia, offensive leucorrhea.

LIMBS: Limbs feel heavy, bruised, sore, as after muscular exertion. Feeling of bruisedness and exhaustion as after influenza. Better from motion.

Sore, tensive pains, especially in right shoulder, in the frontal part of both thighs.

Lumbago, sciatica, burning pains, worse right side, worse sitting, better from pressure, worse beginning and better from continued motion; cannot stay in bed, must get up and walk around at night. Better from warmth, better bending backwards, worse upright position, worse hanging down of legs.

Subacute and chronic arthritis, arthrosis deformans, traumatic arthritis (cf. *Arnica, Symphytum*).

SKIN: Poorly healing skin; styes; furunculosis, oily skin or unclean appearance which soils laundry and linens; itchy, vesicular, herpetic eruptions.

Botanically *Mandragora* belongs to the same family as *Belladonna, Hyoscymus* and *Stramonium,* the family of Solanaceae. It is intensely toxic and fits more the slowly developing and deep seated type of pathology rather than the more acute conditions of *Belladonna,*

Hyoscyamus and *Stramonium.*

Author's Note — This present study of the drug is based on the symptomatology of Mezger's excellent and extensive proving, as well as on the author's own clinical observations and verifications. Mezger stresses that his symptoms were elicited by a preparation of the root. In the author's own experience there seems to be no appreciable difference of action between Mezger's preparation *Mandragora e radice* and our *Mandragora* which is an extract from the leaves.

ARISTOLOCHIA CLEMATIS

This paper introduces a drug into our English Materia Medica which deserves a place foremost among our polychrests. *Aristolochia* is one of the oldest medicinal herbs. It has been used in ancient Egypt, in medieval Europe, as well as by the aborigines of the Americas, particularly against snake bites. The name which the Egyptians gave it is "anti-snake." The name *Aristolochia* is supposed to have been introduced by Paracelsus and means "excellent for labor," thus referring to its relation to the female genital function. It also has had a widespread use in popular medicine as a vulnerary. In animal experiments, carried out by Madaus in Germany, it proved effective against experimental gas gangrene infection. This effect seems to be due to an increase of the defensive forces of the organism since no bacteriostatic action in vitro could be demonstrated. Toxicologically, it causes menorrhagia, abortion, hemorrhagic nephritis, gastroenteritis, fatty degeneration of the liver and internal massive and capillary hemorrhages; it also affects the central nervous system producing nausea, dizziness and convulsions.

Systematic provings upon healthy invididuals were carried out by Julius Mezger of Stuttgart, Germany. The complete Materia Medica of the drug is published in his book *Gesichtete Homeopathische Arzneimittellehre* (Sifted Materia Medica), Karl Haug Verlag, Stuttgart, Germany.

The following presentation is based upon Mezger's symptomatology. Some amplifications are added based upon my own clinical experiences with the drug. Wherever they occur they are specially marked as such by asterisks.

The main directions of action of our drug are:

1. *Urinary tract* (irritation, inflammation, cystitis, pyelitis, polyuria).
2. *The female genital tract* (ovary, anemorrhea, oligomenorrhea, hypomenorrhea, delayed menarche, menopausal arthritis, pregnancy, labor, sterility).
3. *Male genital tract* (prostatitis and epididymitis, G.C.); similar to *Pulsatilla.*
4. *Gastrointestinal tract* (colitis, diarrhea with tenesmus and feeling of unfinishedness); similar to *Mercury.*
5. *Vulnerary* (infected wounds, blisters from mechanical causes — rowing, riding, etc.).
6. *Skin* (chronic and acute eczemas, dermatitis, infections and ulcerations).
7. *Veins* (varicose veins, phlebitis).
8. *Nose and sinuses.*

The medicine strikes us as a hybrid of *Sepia, Pulsatilla* and *Arnica,* if it is permitted at all to express something new, different and unknown in terms of something already familiar. This should not cause us to use the drug as a combination medicine, so to say, when we fail to differentiate between *Sepia* and *Pulsatilla;* remembering those related medicines may help us to grasp the spirit of the new substance by relating it to something already well known. The physical symptoms bear a striking resemblance to *Pulsatilla.* The mentals and the personality type seem nearer to *Sepia.*

Mentals and personality type. In some provers there was depression; in other instances, an existing depression became markedly improved and yielded to a rather cheerful mood particularly before the menstruation. Among my own patients observed so far, the striking observation was the prevalence of extremes of moods, namely either a marked depression or a rather forced or unreasonable exhilaration and cheerfulness, even in alternation. Also found were extreme states of extroversion or introversion in the same person. We may be tempted to classify the *Aristolochia* type as characterized by emotional instability of the manic depressive kind. Tearful depression,* fear of people* (rather than the active spiteful aversion of people), easily offended,* hypersensitive,* lack of self confidence,* complaints of anticipation* (?). They are not easily comforted like *Pulsatilla* but rather inconsolable* and cross* when in the depression, yet not actively aggravated by consolation like *Sepia.** Depression improved with return of suppressed menstruation (after hysterectomy).

General symptoms. Extreme chilliness not better by external heat. Insatiable hunger. Great tiredness and exhaustion or/and alternating with unusual activity and ability to perform — again the manic depressive response pattern. Great exhaustion with dizziness and chilliness not relieved by outer warmth. Extreme hunger in spite of indigestion. Tendency to cold extremities and bunions. *Amenorrhea oligomenorrhea, suppressed menses,* weak and short menses. Poor circulation and local congestion (venous). "Venous type." The *modalities* show a close similarity to the pattern of *Pulsatilla.* The patient is extremely chilly and most local symptoms are better from local heat and worse from cold (particularly the facial neuralgia, toothache and cough). However, the headache and coryza are better from cool air and cool applications. In turn the whole patient desires and is better by cool air, better from motion, better from onset of any discharge; worse before menses and better with onset of menses; the general aggravation is in the morning upon rising and at 2 — 4 A.M. (sleep, cough).

Head — Headaches better open air, cool applications, worse before and *after* menses, better beginning of coryza, worse bending forward.

Eyes — Sensation of scratchiness, burning, lachrymation, worse reading, strong light.

Ears — Tinnitus with otalgia and headaches. Promotes epithelisation after radical operation of middle ear. Acute otitis media.

Nose — Coryza with stuffy nose and headaches, better in cool, open air. Violent headaches better with onset of coryza. Watery coryza with much sneezing, worse 8 — 9 A.M. Nasal polyps with secretion, congestion (local application). Hayfever,* anosmia (?).

Face — Facial neuralgias.

Mouth — Cracked corners of mouth. Herpes labialis. Toothache, apical swelling, worse from cold food, better from warmth.

Throat — Dry throat, sore throat. Yellow coating of tonsils, hoarseness.

Gastrointestinal — Ravenous appetite or loss of appetite. Feeling of squeamishness with empty stomach: faintness, dizziness forcing to lie down. Intense nausea with chilliness. Sour, bitter vomiting; vomiting after sauerkraut, better after milk. Gastritis. Ineffectual desire for stool. Diarrhea with sudden call, so that toilet is barely reached. Virus enteritis with tenesmus; evacuation of mucous without stool. Tenesmus causing rectal prolapse not even better by evacuation of mucous. Chronic enterocolitis with constant rectal pressure soon after evacuation. Diarrhea after each meal. Neurospastic intestinal states.* Emotional,* anticipatory enteritis* and colitis.* Constipation with much flatulence (improved during proving). Bleeding hemorrhoids. The intestinal symptoms are attended by much freezing and chilliness.

Respiratory — Asthma bronchiale.*

Urinary — Frequent desire for urination with pain in bladder and urethra. Painful, frequent urination worse at night. Involuntary dribbling of urine. Enuresis nocturna, cystitis, pyelitis from exposure to cold (soldiers). Sudden pain in kidney area. Albuminuria. Whitish sediment in the urine.

Male genitals — No proving symptoms, but clinically efficacious in prostatitis, epididymitis worse from cold. G.C.

Female genitals — Abdominal cramps before menses. Heaviest dysmenorrhea. Amenorrhea, oligomenorrhea, etc., delayed menarche. Restores menstruation which is too weak or suppressed, even in cases after amputation of uterus. General symptoms better as menses reappear. Amenorrhea due to confinement in prison, camps, flight or travel (*"Lager amenorrhea"*). Amenorrhea of lactation. Menses weaker and shorter. Too early menopause. Leucorrhea, mucous brownish before menses. Mentals and generals worse before menses. Sensation of pain and hardness in left breast. *Itching, voluptuous, of vulva and rectum. Eczema. Swelling of feet and ankles before menses.*

Extremities — Tearing-sticking pains of joints, better at onset of menses or mucous bloody leucorrhea; worse from sewing or knitting.

Menopausal arthroses. Upper arms painful upon pressure. Legs feel heavy like lead. Excessive swelling of the extremities before menses, better onset of menses. Cold extremities.

Varicose veins — Congestion and varicosities of pregnancy. Feeling of tension in varicose veins.

Skin — Pimples and vesicles at various places. Acne* worse before menses; furunculosis.* Extensive dry eczema on neck, arms, etc., itching-burning. Crusty eczema of scalp, labia, vulva, around navel* with intense itching. Erysipeloid eruption on trunk. Dry cracked skin.* Weeping eczemas. Poorly healing skin. Poorly healing wounds; infected wounds. *Blisters from rubbing shoes, rowing, garden work, horseback riding,* etc. Infected blisters from marching (soldiers). Also external injuries from rubbing, pressure and contusions. Chronic ulcers and suppuration of hands and feet. Phlegmon, infected ulcers, dermatitis (10% ointment or 1 — 2 tablespoons of tincture to 500 cc water. For the more acute infections or inflammation rather the watery application).

Prevents infection of fresh wounds and promotes granulation. Painful contusions, burns, frozen extremities. For external applications it seems to be superior to *Calendula.* All sorts of suppurations, septicemia (??).

Temperature regulation — Chilliness over the whole body. Night sweats. Chilliness during menses. Fever with tonsillitis. Cold extremities. *Excessive flashes of heat with perspiration** (menopause).

In routine office work, first consideration is to be given to Aristolochia before any other remedy (unless definitely indicated) in any case of *suppressed or deficient menstruation* (such as usually associated with *Pulsatilla*), as well as in the average case of *cystitis.* As a vulnerary, it seems to be superior to *Calendula.*

Part III
INTO PRACTICE

THE PROBLEM OF SOUL-BODY RELATIONSHIP
IN PRESCRIBING

Long clinical experience has conclusively proven that for the homeopathic treatment, *the characteristic emotional and mental traits of the patient himself* represent the most practical guide towards the selection of the effective medicine, regardless of the kind of clinical illness. In the experiment upon healthy individuals, that medicine must have reproduced not only a state of similar to the physical illness but also a picture of the very emotional and temperamental traits of the patient. This verified empirical rule would imply that the happenings, both on the psycho-emotional, as well as on the organo-physiological level, are among the fundamental elements behind what to us presents itself as disease. In the sense that both psychic and somatic elements are involved, we may be entitled to *look upon most every disorder as a psychosomatic one.* Thus, encouraged by our clinical approach, we may be tempted into the generalization that perchance every such disturbance could be dealt with simply by prescribing a medicine selected on the basis of its psychosomatic similarity; we may expect that medicine always to remove the whole pathology, both psychic and somatic, thus entirely doing away with the need for any psychotherapeutic approaches. Those claims have actually arisen in our midst and they are backed up by many instances of actual therapeutic success in mental diseases as well as in physical disorders with attending emotional symptoms. Yet, alas, life is not so simple that *any one single approach* could encompass the great variety of its phenomena. Every prescriber who is but willing to admit to himself the unpleasant truth may look back upon a goodly number of patients who, with or without the guideposts of marked mental symptoms, have failed to show a lasting response to the similimum, both psycho-emotionally or physically. Particularly, those patients who show a strong emotional background and thus furnish what we would consider the most excellent mental guiding symptoms for exact prescribing not infrequently shock us by this most conspicuous failure of response to the remedy. It is as though *their very psychological impasse presented a barrier to a permanent restoration* of health, ever and again reestablishing pathology after but temporary improvements. Thus, we have to face up to an utterly paradoxical situation. The patient's 'mentals', namely his psychological status, in some cases furnish the foremost leads for a successful therapeutic prescription, yet in other cases these same 'mentals' may be met as obstacles to recovery.

In order to gain a viewpoint from which these contradictory facts can be related to each other as differing aspects of one fundamental phenomenon, a basic consideration of the *interrelation of biologic and psychic functions will have to be attempted.*

When we think of the psyche we frequently tend to explain its function as purely biologic or physiochemical processes. The fact that our psychological dynamism is so strongly motivated by basic instincts as hunger, self-preservation and sexuality, which, in turn, are dependent on hormonal and autonomic nervous activities, supports this attitude. However, in a similar fashion the life processes themselves are interdependent with physical and chemical processes in their turn and yet are not identical with them. Also life cannot be understood by considering it mere complicated chemistry; rather it has to be taken as a qualitatively different basic phenomenon in itself which is *served by chemistry and in turn is dependent on its servant, but not identical with it.* Similarly, psychic processes are interwoven with biologic functions and instincts, but the peculiar human qualities of consciousness, of willing and thinking even against the instinctual demands, are new and distinctive entities. They evolve out of purely animalic life, yet follow different laws of their own. Even with the very psychic processes themselves an analogous further differentiation takes place, as modern depth psychology has shown; the *unconscious and automatic functions become related to an ego center and thus attain an entirely new quality, consciousness.*

Summarizing, we have a peculiar chain of facts: chemistry, as it becomes more complicated, borders into life. Life embodies highly evolved chemistry, but also features an entirely different, new entity which is not chemistry. Biologic functioning, through hormonal and nervous activity, manifests itself in the *instinctual drives* which, on one side, *are highly differentiated biologic functions,* yet in their *psychic differentiation* represent something entirely new and different. Out of the instincts evolves psychic existence culminating in an ego consciousness, a cumulative refinement resulting in the emergence of a new quality. This chain of evolution we see further continued when we realize that even our ego consciousness finds itself confronted with an entity which we feel as continued in our soul, on the one side, and yet, on the other hand, superordinated and above our personal existence and thus different from ourselves. With varying names we have called it ethical, moral, divine, spirit, God immanent (as our highest evolutionary center) and God transcendent (as we experience it apart from ourselves). Thus, evolution seems to advance, on the one side, in a *continuous chain;* on the other hand, by introducing ever *new and diversified variations on different levels.* Each of these is distinct and unique in itself; and yet there are also repetitory patterns, mutual interactions as well as continuous transformations of impulses and energies, from the various levels to each other.

This phenomenon of homogeneous continuity through *discontinuous differentiated entities,* like and yet different, might leave us in a hopeless logical impasse, were it not for the fact that we may profit from the experience of modern physics which successfully dealt with an analogous situation. The nearest example is the *theory of light*, which is considered to be a *continuous, vibratory*, yet at the same time of a *discontinuous, corpuscular nature*, these logically contradictory explanations proving to be mutually complementary in terms of mathematics and practical experience. Applicable to our problem is the fact that long and short waves, infrared, visible light, ultraviolet, Roentgen and radium (gamma) rays *represent different and diversified qualities*, yet, at the same time, *are but variations of the same basic, though, in its essential nature, unknown energy*. Evidencing a continuous chain of phenomenal uniformity which we called spectrum, the various elements of the spectrum nevertheless represent essentially different qualities with different phenomenological laws and effects. Jung[1] commented upon the analogy between the above phenomenology in physics and the findings of analytical psychology, of a spectrum-like relation between *instincts, unconscious psychic elements, conscious psyche and representations of basic spiritual patterns* (referred to as *archetypes*), all of them qualitatively unique entities yet on *different levels*, as it were representing analogous, quasi-repetitory phenomena.

As a practical working hypothesis, we might adopt Jung's symbolic model of a spectral band and extend it *through the whole of psychosomatic existence* from an organic functioning through biochemistry, from biologic life processes through instincts and the realm of the psyche. Just as in the radiation spectrum the visible light is that part which alone is accessible to our direct perception, in the human spectrum, consciousness, like an isolated island, borders on the 'invisible' unconscious elements above and below. As visible light flows into the invisible infrared and thence into short waves and long waves below, and into ultra-violet, leading to high frequency energy above, so the "visible", conscious psyche flows *"below" into the unconscious of the instincts* which lead on to biology and chemistry, and *"above" into the emotional, ethical and religious experience leading into the realm of the spirit*. In a simplified way we thus may consider the physiologic functioning the bottom layer of the unconscious.

However, the human spectrum is not static and two dimensional but moves on in never-ending evolutional changes which include the space (central versus peripheral manifestations) as well as time factor (coexistence of past factors as well as future trends in a given symptom picture). This fascinating quality of *four dimensionality* would, however, exceed the limit of our subject were we to discuss it now. The evolutional changes are characterized by slow progressions and regressions, as well as by rather tempestuous concentrations of energy,

159

alternating with phases of comparative calm. Ever and again, there is an emergence of what we may liken to storm centers of accumulated energy with subsequent release of tension, when a forward step is being enforced or the strength of the impulse is stalled or has spent itself. To our subjective experience, such storm centers present themselves as physiologic or psychologic disturbances. Their symptoms depend upon the area of the 'spectrum' in which they stir as well as upon their intensity, which results in various degrees of extension into the adjoining regions.

Like in a model experiment, we can study the peculiar spread of the disturbance of an energetic field by watching what happens when a stone drops into the water. The intensity of the spreading wave ripples diminishes with distance. When the spread is blocked by an obstacle, the waves are reflected; turning back, they add to the original disturbance and confuse its pattern. In analogy, the energetic disturbance, created by a storm center in the human 'spectrum', tends to spread into the adjoining areas in ratio to the intensity of the central field, diminishing with the degree of spread. When the *extension meets a barrier the energetic flow is reflected; turning back, it adds to the original disturbance, changing its pattern and bringing forth expressions* in different directions. In this way, the empirically well-known symptomatology of suppression is accounted for.

For instance, a 'storm center' situated in the 'area' of *hormonal and autonomous central regulation will affect the directly adjoining field or organ functions and biochemistry* perhaps giving rise to circulatory or rheumatic disorders. The "upward" extension would affect the *instinctual sphere* and hence produce emotional symptoms, typical perhaps of menopause or puberty. According to our hypothesis, a blocking of the extension in one direction should intensify the flow of disorder into the opposite one. Actually, we have observed that thwarted organic expressions (stopped discharges or rashes, removal of organs, etc.) may often be followed by more serious disorder, even by mental disturbances. Conversely, *repressions of instinctual conflicts which prevent their extension into consciousness, lead to disturbances "lower down"* in the organic sphere, as confirmed by the psychosomatic literature of recent years.

Obviously, the optimal therapeutic approach depends upon the correct *diagnosis of the 'location' of the focus of the turbulence* and, secondly, upon the understanding of how the various therapeutic methods affect those different areas of the 'spectrum'. The homeopathic provings seem to suggest that the potentized medicine exerts its main effect upon the 'lower' part where *chemistry and vitality meet.* From there, a further downward spread of its action affects *gross chemistry and organic structure;* the upward extension of its energy reaches into the *instincts, desires, aversions, temperamental traits and states of mind.* The more material effect of allopathic dosage, chemical and mechanical therapy (infusions, surgery, etc.) centers even further "down" towards gross chemistry and substance structure. The psychotherapeutic approach, in turn, acts directly upon the "upper" sphere where our consciousness interplay with the unconscious instincts on the one side, and the unconscious spiritual impulses on the other side. Its downward extension, through instinctual and hormonal nervous regulation, may affect the physiologic and biochemic organ functioning.

Probably the main difficulty in diagnosing the central focus of the energetic disturbance is accounted for by the fact that the patient's awareness of symptoms is determined by the 'wave ripples' which happen to reach his little island of consciousness. In registering these we cannot be sure, at first, where they originated and whether all the waves actually reached our observation point. Many a storm may be subjectively asymptomatic by not reaching our consciousness island at all; many messages are received only indirectly from secondary manifestations. For instance, a condition manifesting, let us say, as choleocystopathy may, in one instance, be the extension of a constitutionally inherited hormonal, secretory and autonomic nervous imbalance and thus require a *constitutional medical approach.* In another case, the same picture may arise from an unconscious repressed psychological conflict situation of which, at first, we perceive only the organo-physiologic reverberations. In turn, one case with predominantly mental disturbances may represent a *deadlocked psychological* conflict; another one with similar symptoms may arise through *organic imbalances.*

At this point, two short case histories are offered which, by their comparative similarity, illustrate the difficulty of deciding for the best therapeutic approach.

Mrs. M.L., age 49, for 10 years suffering from weekly attacks of severe migraine. The attacks are left-sided, with pains that feel like piercing the eye, attended by a globus sensation in the throat, abdominal cramps and vomiting. The patient is irritable, over-sensitive, easily offended, cries easily, feels worse before the period, worse from exposure to the sun, worse from approaching thunderstorms, chilly but better in open air and craves sweets. She is married to a much older, very fickle man by whom she is utterly dominated and seemingly not too well treated. Her emotional attitude being of a still rather adolescent character, she cannot cope with her situation, except by fits of rage and despair. Under *Sulphur* and *Sepia* there is a general constitutional improvement along with prompt control of intercurrent acute disturbances; yet, over a period of six years, the migraine tendency persists. At the end of this time, psychoanalytic therapy was

161

instituted. As she becomes aware that in her marriage relation she unconsciously still lived her childhood and adolescent pattern towards her also *quite domineering father* and succeeds in acquiring a more mature emotional outlook, she succeeds in holding her own in her present relation. A new *modus vivendi* is established in her marital situation and now, for a year, there has been neither any recurrence of migraine nor of any of the other frequent acute disorders that formerly plagued her.

Miss J.C., age 24. Attacks of unexplainable compulsive terror and apprehension, seizing and almost paralyzing her when walking in the street. Feels as though she would faint, with cold perspiration, heart palpitations and trembling all over. She is irritable, impatient, cannot cry, feels better during her relation to her fiance whom she thinks she does not love; however, neither is she able to deny herself to him or to effect a break. She can't say "No" to a man. Also, here, an immature emotional attitude is confirmed by her dependence on a domineering father with whom she still lives and from whom she cannot tear herself loose. *Sepia* 1M., single dose, completely removes the, to her, so threatening symptom complex; this in spite of the still persisting personal difficulty. For several months there has been no recurrence, though, in the face of the general background, there are doubts about the future. Here, apparently, a basic, hormonal autonomic nervous liability was responsible for the excessively dysbalancing effect of a fairly average personal problem, thus justifying a medical approach. An understanding of this intricate and contradictory soul-body relationship may protect us from the mistake of considering a case incurable or of changing the remedy when a correct prescription does not seem to work. The difficulty may simply lie in the fact that one particular approach has, for the time at least, *reached its limit of practical applicability.*

Undoubtedly, our understanding is still extremely fragmentary and our auxiliary hypothesis may perhaps appear rather complicated and far fetched. We ought to remember, however, that our position is similar to that of physics, in respect to nuclear research, where we have progressed to that point where the utterly abstract and complicated findings cannot be made clear except by means of structural models which are but pictorial analogies or symbols. Also the atom model does not represent an actually observable reality, but, like our 'spectrum', is the best possible way of expressing something unperceivable, by means of a comparison or symbolic representation.

Such are our stumbling attempts, also in medicine to proceed from a static, mechanistic approach to one that reckons in terms of *systems and fields*. Physics has outgrown its mechanistic childhood. So has, in part at least, the still comparatively recent science of psychology. It is time, also for medicine now to shoulder the difficult task and free itself from the shackles of the mechanistic thinking which was the heritage of the nineteenth century.

[1]C.G. Jung: Der Geist der Psychologie. Eranos Jahrbuch, 1946, Rhein Verlag, Zuerich.

PROBLEMS OF CHRONIC PRESCRIBING

Today, the efficiency of medical treatment is generally measured by its success in extreme conditions. This standard, necessarily, applies only either to acute illness or to terminal conditions like cancer, etc. An advocate of Homeopathy finds himself immediately confronted with the question if Homeopathy can cure cancer, leukemia or meningitis and whether we have anything to match modern chemotherapy and the antibiotics. Moreover, while admitting the efficiency of Homeopathy in acute illness, as well as in the palliation of incurable degenerative conditions, many a superficial inquirer may still feel that the use of penicillin in pneumonia or of opiates for the palliation of cancer is simpler and therefore preferable.

Yet, the fact is overlooked that many things incurable could well be prevented. And in the field of preventative therapeutics, Homeopathy is simply and absolutely without equal. Beyond the general principles of sanitation and the rather doubtful blessings of massive vaccination the orthodox approach can not even claim to have made any beginning of effective disease prevention.

It is claimed that one out of every four persons dies of cancer. In New York City two out of every thousand are registered cases of tuberculosis. How many homeopathic patients, under steady chronic treatment for conditions other than these did during, let us say, 5 or 10 years develop cancer or tuberculosis? According to the statistical probability, at least a certain percentage of people observed over this length of time should have developed these conditions. Yet, the files of any homeopath who engages in systematic chronic work will reveal an astoundingly, out of proportion, low statistical incidence of newly-developing degenerative illness among his constitutionally treated chronic cases.

Moreover, one forgets too easily that the absence of acute illness does not yet mean good health. Whereas many acute cases get well by themselves, regardless of treatment, for the majority of chronic ailments allopathy knows of no therapy at all except surgery. All of this is to show that both from the angle of prevention as well as of treatment the chronic constitutional work is the very core of the homeopathic contribution to Medicine which is absolutely unique and unrivaled.

On the other hand, the handling of a chronic patient is beset with difficulties and pitfalls which make it the most difficult chapter of case management. Some of these most vexing problems are to be discussed in this paper. We start from the premise that the case has been properly taken and studied and that the remedy was carefully selected.

Our difficulty arises when the apparently well chosen remedy does not live up to our expectations but either:

1. Fails completely to cause any improvement.
2. Relieves only partly.
3. Does not hold for a sufficiently long time.
4. Fails upon repetition, though the symptoms are still the same.

1. If the prescription has no effect at all, obviously the remedy, although chosen on the basis of the best available evidence, was not really indicated, at least not at the given moment. By this last modification it is implied that, sometimes, a remedy which correctly covers the case has to have its way prepared by another, related one. We shall return to this point later. Our first reaction to the failure of our prescription, however, must be to question its absolute correctness. If the remedy was really carefully chosen upon proper study and evaluation of the symptomatic material, we may assume that this material itself was deficient and did not encompass the complete symptom totality.

What is really meant with symptom totality? It is not necessarily the greater number of symptoms that make the totality but the evidence of those symptoms, even if they be few in number, which are characteristic of a drug proving and distinguish its peculiar sphere of action from similar ones. Thus, in designating the symptom totality, we make a *qualitative selection* from the available material, being guided in our evaluation by our knowledge and understanding of the Materica Medica. On the other hand, the patient's totality is, usually, only a fraction of the remedy's totality, as we studied it. For instance, in the study of *Lachesis* its totality consists of the seasonal aggravation, the aggravation after sleep, from tight clothes, stuffy rooms, suppressed discharges, of its loquacity, jealousy, etc., along with its peculiar sensations and localities. Yet, in a patient we may need only aggravation in the fall, after sleep, and jealousy, three symptoms in all, to indicate *Lachesis,* and *Lachesis* alone, regardless of the nature of the ailment. Expressed in different words: The patient's totality need not consist of *all* characteristic symptoms of the drug, but the drug must have all of the patient's peculiar and characteristic symptoms. Still, we may take our case with attention to an endless number of details, which may be relatively unimportant, since they may be shared by too many remedies, and yet overlook or disregard a little symptom, meaningless from the clinical standpoint, but peculiar to a few drugs only and thus indispensable for the charting of the correct totality.

A case for illustration: Mrs. M., 57 years. Pain in right side of the chest, remaining after pleurisy. Chronic appendicitis, illeocecal tenderness and constriction. No appetite, feeling of fullness and nausea. Constipation and distension. Rightsided headaches. Feeling as if the abdominal organs would fall out. Great weakness and lassitude with gradual, steady loss of weight. Depression, indefinite fears and restlessness, yet satisfied to be alone. Worse in late afternoon and evening, from pressure of clothes, better from warm applications. General lack of vital heat. *Lycopodium* 200. to 10M gave some relief but never was able to overcome the trouble completely. *Sepia* which is strongly suggested by the symptoms made no impression. After several months of relatively unsatisfactory progress the patient attended a lecture on the importance of observing even minor symptoms and subsequently reported to the doctor that at times she had fine cracks at the tip of her nose. Under this symptom Kent lists only *Alumina* in highest and *Carbo animalis* in the lowest degree. Yet, once thought of, low vitality in old people, desire to be alone, sadness, reflectiveness, anxiety in the evening, stiches remaining after pleurisy, weak digestion with flatulence, cracks at the tip of the nose do add up to *Carbo animalis* and *Carbo animalis* gave the aid which *Lycopodium* had failed to produce.

The cracks on the nose pointed in the new direction but only together with the other characteristic symptoms was the prescription determined. If the cracks alone were made the basis for the selection, one would be guilty of keynote prescribing.

Often our remedy selection will be incorrect because the miasmatic factor was not considered. Strictly speaking, a history of Syphilis, G.C., Tuberculosis or Malaria must be considered a part of the symptom totality. In a proving, the symptoms develop not only in space, that is, simultaneously, upon different parts, but also in a timely sequence. Therefore we must take into consideration that what is available of symptoms at the time we take the case, represents only a spatial distribution. In order to avail ourselves of the distribution in time, we must carefully check the past history and perhaps even forecast the likely future development, if unchecked, for instance when prescribing for what we should recognize as a cancerous diathesis. Any history of the above conditions, therefore, should be considered as if present at the given moment and included in the prescribing material.

A patient with occupational eczema due to allergy to hairdyes is remembered, who, while giving a perfect picture of *Sulphur,* failed to respond, until it was preceded by *Thuja, Medorrhinum,* and *Tuberculinum.* This case had a history of a G.C. infection as well as of an arrested Tuberculosis.

Often no miasmatic history can be obtained. Being reasonably sure that our presribing was thorough and careful, not superfically routine, we may deduce the presence of the miasmatic factor from the very failure of this seemingly correct prescription itself. In this rare instance we choose the remedy on a basis of pure reasoning, without symptomatic guide.

Mrs. T., 55, bronchial asthma. Very irritable; the asthma started with the menopause, is worse at night and wakes her from sleep, worse in damp weather, in warm weather and in the fall. Intolerant to tight clothing. *Lachesis* 200. — 10M gives splended relief for 6 months, then stops working. No new or different symptoms, except some vaginal itching. In spite of absolutely no evidence of any venereal history a miasmatic obstacle is postulated and *Medorrhinum* 200. single dose given. There has been no need for any further prescription for this condition for the last twelve months.

2. Sometimes only a partial relief follows the administration of the remedy. Such a case we will judge upon whether or not Hering's postulates for a cure are being followed (symptoms moving from above downwards, from inside out and from more to less vital parts). Whenever this pattern is adhered to and the patient feels better, mentally and as a whole, our prescription was correct, though some of his peripheral symptoms may even be worse. If, however, vital parts remain unimproved, though peripheral symptoms disappear or the patient, as a whole, fails to improve, we should assume that our prescription was only partly similar and a more suitable remedy has to be looked for.

Mrs. G., 55 yrs. Grand mal epilepsy, excessive varicosities of both legs with multiple varicose ulcers, gradually decompensating heart failure. Patient is heavy, plethoric, with venous stasis all over the body, flushes of heat, sore bruised sensation. *Arnica* 30. Excellent improvement of the feet but increased frequency and intensity of the epileptic spells which take on a threatening aspect. Medication discontinued. Epilepsy better, feet worse. *Arnica* renewed. Feet better, epilepsy worse. Case restudied, *Sulphur* 200. given. At first epilepsy better, feet worse, then everything gradually but steadily improving. Such a case demonstrates that a partly similar homeopathic prescription may act suppressively in the same way as an allopathic drug or ill-advised surgery.

A special problem arises when we have to prescribe for a case which exhibits only very few symptoms. Hahnemann points out *(Organon* 175 — 184) that in such an instance the best selected remedy, if it cannot affect a complete cure, since it is only partly suited to the case, will be instrumental in arousing the patient's vitality, so as to bring out more symptoms which can form the basis for a better second prescription. According to my own experience this "vital reaction" not infrequently is quite stormy; the patient passes through apparently more serious trouble after the treatment was instituted than before. In very deep-seated disorders months or even years of temporarily quite violent suffering may ensue after the dormant state has been roused into activity. The doctor as well as the patient ought to be aware of this possibility in order not to lose heart and to avoid suppressive palliation, though surgical help may be necessary at times when irreversibly devitalized tissue has to be removed. If we patiently continue prescribing through this phase, a very satisfactory general improvement usually follows the crisis. It is different when the paucity we prescribe upon is only an apparent one. If there are sufficient symptoms to make a good prescription, yet they are overlooked by us, our prescription will not arouse a low vitality; there was no need for a stimulus to produce symptoms and our incomplete prescription is just incorrect. There will be either no response at all or a suppressive one, confusing the symptoms and lowering the patient's vitality instead of arousing it. Unless a very acute condition demands an antidotal prescription it is best to choose one's remedy on a more careful re-evaluation of the original state, prior to the wrong remedy.

3. The response to our prescription should last for a certain length of time before a new dose becomes necessary. When a repetition seems required too soon we should become suspicious. Yet, exactly how long should one dose act? No hard and fast rules can be laid down since there are many factors which can affect the duration of action. The most important ones are: Age, the type of the personality as well as of the disorder, the presence of obstacles to a cure, the potency prescribed, whether it is the first or a later prescription and finally the kind of remedy itself.

Children seem to have a much more rapid rate of life and metabolic functioning than older people. Biologically speaking, we might say that a minute is as full to them as an hour to us, while to the older person an hour seems only like a minute (to eternity a century is but a day). In children this more intense life activity reflects itself, among other things, in a higher respiratory and circulatory rate and a higher body temperature, while the intellectual activities remain relatively in the background. Conversely, in a more advanced age, the forces of life and metabolism appear to be converted into the faculties of consciousness with a resulting slowing down and lowering of the biologic and regenerative rhythmus.

Thus, a remedy effect, although of the same duration, in terms of what we may call "biological time," appears to be consumed more quickly in the child and more slowly in the old person, in terms of our "standard" time. Consequently, children often require more frequent prescriptions and older people less frequent ones, compared to the average adult.

The very same concept of "biological time" can be applied to the diverse clinical conditions and personality types. The faster the biologic activity the more quickly the remedy effect will appear as well as vanish. Feverish conditions often require hourly repetitions; in the most acute emergencies one may have to repeat even every few minutes. The gradually developing chronic states respond slowly and bear only infrequent prescriptions.

An analogous pattern emerges when we compare the various consti-tutional types. A choleric fast-living person requires more remedies during the same time span than a torpid or phlegmatic one. Since the remedies themselves are fitted to personalities and conditions we will not be surprised to find that such drugs as *Aconite* or *Nux vomica,* matching choleric types or most acute fevers, are usually, though not always, of quicker yet shorter action than let us say *Lycopodium* or *Hydrastis* which are adapted to slow, cautious people or states of debilitation, chronicity and old age.

The deeper the constitutional layer affected, the slower is the biological pace in which it moves and the less frequently is a repetition demanded and tolerated. The depth of the remedy therefore also suggests the length of its duration. Most mineral remedies are deeper and therefore slower than herb and animal drugs. Likewise the higher the potency the deeper and consequently the longer is its effect.

Sometimes, the first prescription acts only for a relatively short time, paving the way, as it were, for the following dose, which, though in the same potency, may act much longer. Probably because of this experience Hahnemann developed his method of plussing which in some cases of delayed response proves extremely useful.

On the average, the first prescription of a 200. may hold only for a week but the second or third doses should act for about a month and the higher dynamizations even longer. If, however, 50M or a CM which, reached by a step raising of the potencies, should act for several months, fails even to approximate the alloted time span, we have to consider the possibility of an obstacle to recovery or some irreversible tissue breakdown; if those are unlikely we should question the correctness of our prescription. The case of chronic appendicitis, mentioned before, which superficially bore the aspects of *Lycopodium,* required repetitions of *Lycopodium every 7—10 days. Carbo animalis,* on the other hand, given on the better evaluation of the totality, gave a response of several months to the single dose.

4. When a remedy has caused a satisfactory general response but fails to act again, even in higher or lower potency, when demanded again by the patient's condition, the need for a new prescription arises. Very rarely will a chronic case be completely cured by but one remedy. However, merely a change of symptoms does not justify a different remedy as long as the patient's general condition improves and the change follows Hering's direction of cure. Only if the general state does not improve and the same remedy, even in a different potency, fails to evoke a response, is a new prescription called for, and even though the symptoms should be the same as before. It is necessary that we clearly understand this paradox: changed symptoms may not

justify a change of remedy (the general progress being satisfactory). Yet the same symptoms may demand a different remedy (if the general condition fails to improve upon repetition).

But how are we to choose a new remedy while the symptoms on which we based our first, now voided, prescription are still the same? In this dilemma the knowledge of complementary relationships will help a great deal. We must not fall into the mistake of prescribing a drug routinely, just because it is listed as complementary. We will give only our first consideration to the complementary drugs in our restudying of the case. Often then we will find that the leading symptoms are shared by several remedies from among which we may choose the most closely indicated one. In the case of chronic appendicitis, mentioned before, after *Carbo animalis* had completed its work and did not hold any longer, *Sepia* was required on the basis of: weakness, depression, fear, desire to be alone, worse evenings, worse pressure clothes, better warmth; all these symptoms are to be found under *Carbo animalis* and *Lycopodium* as well.

Boeninghausen's repertory has a little-used section on relationships of remedies which is especially useful for this purpose. Under the heading of the last successful but now failing remedy one can select the most closely related drugs by applying the method of repertorial analysis.

Mrs. A., 41 yrs. Manic depressive state. Recently dismissed from a state institution where she spent about 6 months of the depressive phase. At present slightly manic but fairly reasonable and aware of her predicament. Dictatorial, irritable, aversion to company, difficult concentration, sadness before menses, menses scanty and too short, obese, can't stand being touched, lack of vital heat. Choking in the throat, desire for salt, dizziness, deep sleep. Numbness of upper extremities. Dazed during the day. *Conium* 200. – 10M gives good response for 5 months then fails upon repetition. *Calcarea carbonica, Natrum muriaticum* unavailing. Upon repertorising *Conium* still appears to lead. Boenninghausen's section on related remedies is consulted under *Conium.*

Repertorizing the groupings of mind, sleep and dreams and sensations 16 remedies emerge of which *Cannabis Indica, Opium* and *Phosphoric acid* were studied. Neither of these had come out by the Kent method. Upon additional questioning the patient gave a history of previous exhaustion by excessive drinking and overwork, which decided for *Phosphoric acid.* Absolute and complete recovery. The patient is still being observed, after 4 years. She meanwhile quite suddenly lost her husband and not only took the tremendous shock without losing her balance but has assumed the whole responsibility for supporting herself and her children, by teaching.

Not infrequently, after the complementary drug has carried on, for a while, from where the first prescription left off, it also ceases to be effective. Again a different, related drug will have to be found or the patient may revert to the original remedy. Some cases seem to go in a steady circle or spiral, following 3 — 4 remedies in cycles of several repetitions each time, and reverting to the first one again when the round is complete, yet steadily improving during this sequence. In other instances, a very obviously indicated remedy will not act at all, unless preceded by a different related one, which apparently removes a basic constitutional obstacle.

Mr. T., 38 yrs. Chronic sinusitis, yellow heavy nasal discharge; tall, thin intellectual type, irritable, cross and critical; easily fatigued, heavy-staining perspiration. Worse at night, in cold damp weather, chilly but craving open air. *Sulphur* unavailing; *Silica* brings gratifying relief but stops working after 2 months. Under *Tuberculinum* progress is resumed for 5 months, then it also fails. *Syphilinum* now gives the most pronounced reaction, holding for about 8 months. Now *Silica, Tuberculinum, Phosphorus, Sulphur, Hepar* are tried with no effect. Finally under *Aurum sulph.* progress is resumed (better open air, worse cold night, critical, aversion to company and the *Sulphur* type with the *syphilitic miasm*). Four months later the patient reverted to *Silica* again, thus completing the cycle; yet after 6 months of progress under *Silica, Sulphur* is demanded and though not effective in the beginning, now brings about a spectacular response.

Miss K., 10 yrs. Tall, thin, slow. Red rimmed eyes, subfebrile states, leucorrhea, heavy perspiration, underweight, desiring highly seasoned food. *Sulphur* does not act until preceded for about 1 year by *Calcarea phosphorica* and occasional doses of *Tuberculinum*. Interestingly enough, in the repertorial analysis *Sulphur, Phosphorus* and *Calcarea* were leading, neither of which would elicit any response in the beginning. Only by combining *Calcarea* and *Phosphorus* into the salt, a reaction could be started which paved the way for the final, constitutional remedy, *Sulphur*.

Cases of this kind, of course, offer the most baffling problems to the prescriber. Sometimes a slight shift of the accentuation of some mentals or modalities might give us a hint in what direction to move. Where there is absolutely no change in the symptom picture while our best remedy refuses to act upon repetition, our ingenuity is put to a serious test. An intimate knowledge of Materia Medica coupled with careful use of the repertory plus sufficient time for restudying the case will always be the indispensable premise for our decision. However, when the scales are absolutely evenly balanced, pointing with equal strength to several drugs, none of which can claim any preponderance, an objective method of picking the remedy is asked for. The most likely drugs can be tested upon the patient's autonomic reflexes, as described by Stearns (Stearns and Evia: *A New Synthesis,* 1942).

The testing of the pupil or Kinesiology reflexes can be easily made part of the office routine. With some experience it will greatly enhance the accuracy of our prescribing.

There are, of course, many more situations which may pose quite perplexing problems. The homeopath, when he fails, can seldom find comfort in the common medical attitude that science knows no answer for the condition which defies him. The range of possibilities, inherent in Homeopathy, is so boundless, that as individuals we can not but measure up poorly against it. On the other hand, for this very reason, we never need to accept our failures as unalterable. Constant striving can still narrow the range of our failures, though forever the old Latin proverb remains true: *Ars longa vita brevis.* Art is long, but short our life.

PSYCHOSOMATICS

The so called psychogenesis of at least some states of physical disorder has been adequately established during the last few decades. The homeopathic provings have shown that specific physiological imbalances are attended by changes in emotional equilibrium which show a certain broad specificity for certain drug induced disorders.

The homeopathic prescriber has learned to use the mentals (actually alterations of the affect responses for most of them pertain to the emotions, not to the mind) as aids in finding the simillimum in the treatment of physical conditions, ordinarily classified as somatic disorders. This is based on the rationale that the somatic derangement of the proving is attended by emotional alterations which operate in demonstrable functional unity with the emotions.

Yet, how about the so called psychogenic disorder? How does the simillimum work in these cases and what directions, if any, can be given for case management in the treatment of neuroses, psychoses and their attending physical symptoms? Where is the line to be drawn between prescribing a remedy and prescribing psychotherapy? In this paper a short discussion of this question is to be attempted, based on a few typical clinical examples chosen more or less at random from my practice in which I use both the simillimum, as well as analytical psychotherapy.

Case 1. An elderly lady with a weeping eczema spreading over both feet, legs, thighs, violently itching and crusty, worse from washing and heat. Constitutionally this patient was a typical *Sulphur* case, heavy, fat, sweaty with oily skin and her various acute and chronic symptoms had well responded to *Sulphur* up to now. Hence, *Sulphur* seemed clearly indicated but equally clearly it did no good whatsoever. A few stumbling prescribing efforts were made but were soon given up for lack of any symptoms pointing to anything beyond the obvious *Sulphur*. Instead I talked to her about her personal life. At once it came out that prior to the onset of her skin condition, her sister had been committed to a State Hospital. This caused her profound shame and grief; while hesitantly telling me this she could not restrain her tears. *Natrum muriaticum* was at once given; in spite of her obesity, 2 doses 200 and 1M sufficed to clear the condition. While one does not think at once of *Natrum muriaticum* in eczema conditions, or for that matter, in obese people, it nevertheless has raw eczema to a high degree and particularly leads in ailments following mortification and grief.

Case 2. By way of contrast I remember a middleaged woman with pronounced quite disfiguring acne of the face. She ran consistently on

Sepia and *Natrum muriaticum* for her various constitutional and acute ailments. Everything responded promptly to the remedy but her acne would not budge. Because of increasing pressure of personal problems, analytic psychotherapy was started. Working with her dreams brought to light a strong unconscious concern and feeling of shame about being Jewish. During her teens she had strongly suffered from the prevailing discrimination and felt she ought to hide the fact that she was Jewish when applying for jobs in order to "save face." At that time the facial eruption began and persisted for the next 20 years in spite of the simillimum, until the repressed feelings were brought to light. Then only, without any further prescribing, the facial eruption improved. For other intercurrent conditions *Sepia* and *Natrum muriaticum* still remained the required remedies.

Case 3. A young man, age 18 complains about consistently recurring swelling of his throat preventing him from swallowing, making him choke. The angle of the jaw feels swollen and painful. There are sensations as of protuberances on the skull and he feels ridges appearing on the skull. He also feels as though his pelvic bones had changed shape and structure, as though his energy were fading away; in spite of increasing exhaustion, he cannot sleep, he is afraid of being incurably ill. There were absolutely no physical findings to substantiate his symptoms; we deal with a severe anxiety neurosis here. Previous prescribing by experienced colleagues had been in vain; indeed there seemed to be no remedy in sight to me either, to fit that case. I had a two hour interview with him in the course of which, a dream brought to light what really bothered him. He felt threatened by his strong sexual urges which he was determined to hold in check rigidly. The more rigidly he repressed them the more they grew and tortured him. Turning his mind away from them produced the anxiety syndromes which became projected upon the previously presented symptoms, typically again in the language of body symbolism affecting pelvic area and head (the two areas in conflict) and the dysphagia depicting the vain attempt to "swallow" his conflict. Yet, for prescribing, these symptoms were useless. The symptoms actually chosen, the mentals on the basis of what the analysis of his dream revealed, were: ailments of shame, amorous dreams and illusions, enlargements of parts of the body, sleepy but cannot sleep, oversensitivity, spasms of the throat, violent sexual excitement. The remedy is *Opium,* administered in 200 and 1M potencies. Together with a thorough "talking it out" of the necessity for giving the needs of the body their place the situation was resolved.

Case 4. The next case is a woman in a serious climacteric depression with panicky fear of any responsibility, crying and despair whenever any responsibility — guests, entertaining, etc., have to be accepted.

She felt like running away, hiding from everything. The patient was a *Phosphorus* type, refined, wellbred, oversensitive, quiet, retiring and disciplined never to show the emotions which now got the better of her. There were also serious rheumatic symptoms and chronic eczemas. The prescribing results were indifferent and finally she had to be hospitalized in profound stupor; shock therapy was used. After that she returned to me. She was a bit less depressed than during her worst days but was in the dazed state usually to be found after shock therapy. The attempt at analysis did not get us very far. But at least it was possible to bring to her, as well as her doctors, awareness of the fact that underneath the surface of an oversensitive refined cultured and overdisciplined person there smoldered a volcano of violent temper, resentment and vicious hostility. The volcano-like temperament points to *Magnesium.* The refined surface amounts to *Phosphorus.* *Magnesium phosphoricum* in the whole potency range from 200 to CM over long periods along with what little insights she had gained enabled her to function and face at least a minimum of her responsibilities.

The last case shows an interesting combination of determining modalities. This was a maiden lady living a withdrawn virtuous life taking care of her niece, who was quite a hellion and lived it up with men and drink. Through hovering and worrying over her problem child, her niece, our patient experienced in a vicarious fashion what her own life had denied her. As she approached the change of life the "bad" niece suddenly up and left her and got married in another part of the country. The patient's life suddenly having become empty and at the same time passing through climacterium a serious emotional imbalance ensued; she became depressed and slipped on the street and broke the neck of the femur; this, following surgical intervention and about two months hospitalization, produced a persistent lameness. This was her form of nervous breakdown, we may say; frequently accidents occur as unconscious attempts at suicide. The residual lameness was better from warmth, worse from rising but better from continued motion: it slowly responded to *Sepia* which had also formerly helped her in many conditions. But now, as the menstrual cycle dwindled, a most annoying cystopathy developed, with intensely painful micturation more of a spastic than inflammatory nature. Worse before menses and better at the onset of menstrual flow. Her emotional state was now of irritable depression. Urinary pathology not infrequently develops in women in consequence of repressed emotional, especially sexual tension. In terms of general symptoms we have now a picture of depressive irritability, oligomenorrhea, worse before and better at the onset of menses, general chilliness, better from warmth, better from continued motion especially in the open air, emotional and sexual repression, complaints of climacterium, traumatic arthritis, urinary irritation.

One finds oneself wavering between *Lachesis* and *Pulsatilla,* perhaps with a dash of *Arnica;* for neither of them fully fits the picture. The full remedy totality is to be found in *Aristolochia clematis:* depressive irritability, menopause and amenorrhea, genitourinary and traumatic pathology, often traumatic cystitis, worse before and better at onset of menses and free secretions, arthritis, rheumatism, better from menstruation, chilly, better from heat, from motion, better in the open air.

I have selected a number of cases of obvious psychosomatic interaction which in the therapeutic response showed all possible reaction from full refractoriness to the simillimum, instead requiring psychotherapy, to prompt response to the remedy without any psychotherapeutic elucidation. Between these extreme poles are cases where response to the remedy is unsatisfactory unless psychological exploration takes place. The psychological exploration confronts the physician with insights into psychodynamics essential for proper remedy selection or directly helps the patient by relieving those emotional tensions which block the response to the remedy.

There is no rational way to arrive at a prima facie differential diagnosis between somatogenic and psychogenic disorder. The practical way is "ex remedio" whichever approach happens to help.

In our last case, is the depression somatogenic due to menopause or is the menopausal pathology psychogenic? Is the cystitis of traumatic origin or are fracture and cystitis psychogenic? Are the body hallucinations of our youngsters psychogenic or are obsessive states and puberty depressions somatogenic? Is the body the deepest level of the unconscious or the psyche the highest level of biological differentiation? One may go on splitting hair indefinitely, failing to realize that the whole question rests on an *a priori* dualistic splitting into body and mind, of what essentially is a functional unit manifesting to our sensory experience as though dualistically separated.

Tertium non datur; the inexplicable individual totality incarnated in body and soul, Paracelsus' Archeus, the "subtle" body of the mystic, or whatever else you may wish to call it, is not directly observable. It may be described or circumscribed but not defined.

The problem of psychosomatics arises merely in the question of the *most practical management* of an individual situation, namely whether the remedy or the psychological exploration or a combination of both are likely to be most effective. A remedy is, of course, simpler, less time consuming and cheaper than psychotherapy. And yet where the latter seems obviously indicated it is wasteful to spend one's time and the patient's money to work out a remedy which has no chance to help.

From my own experience I have come through the years to a way of prognostic differentiation which I would call the *law of modalities*. I have taken the nature, preponderance or absence of modalities, to indicate the direction of therapeutic management and likely prognosis. A preponderance of mental and emotional modalities points to the necessity of psychotherapy whereas the preponderance of physical modalities makes me expect more of the remedy. The less of *any* modalities, the poorer the prognosis either way. Please take note that I say *modalities* not *mental symptoms*. A case may have many mental symptoms and yet few or no emotional modalities. Modalities are not merely characteristics or symptoms or concomitants but are *conditions of amelioration and aggravation*. They indicate the fixedness or changeableness, hence, the responsiveness of the organism and of the pathology. They indicate the position of the therapeutic problem in the total life process, liability, over-responsiveness or hypersensitivity or stability, lack of responsiveness or insensitivity. Midway between these two poles stands adequate therapeutic responsiveness and the capacity to growth and change through trial and suffering.

Preponderance of physical modalities makes me look for a remedy; preponderance of emotional modalities makes me tend to explore the unconscious psychological background. Too few modalities make me shake my head. The mental symptoms and characteristics are to be considered when and if owing to presence of physical modalities a remedy is to be selected. Hence, the mental *symptoms* in differentiation to the mental *modalities* do not help to determine if a remedy is to be used but *what* remedy if any at all. For instance the depressive wicked temper of *Lachesis* will call for the drug only when the patient's ailments are made worse also by sleep, season, etc. If the temperamental state per se brings about the aggravations without physical responsiveness, in other words, when we have only a *Lachesis* temper and pathology but not many biological signs of *Lachesis* like physical responsiveness I would not expect too much or too lasting an effect from the remedy. Then the appeal to consciousness and realization would have to have priority.

The most important medicines among the 82 which Kent lists under IMPATIENCE are: *Acon., Ars., Aur., Bry., Calc., Cham., Coloc., Hep., Ign., Iod., Kali c., Lach., Lyc., Med., Nat. m., Nux v., Plat., Psor., Puls., Rhus tox., Sep., Sil., Staph., Sulf.*

Arg. nitr. does not appear in Kent but certainly should be added to the list, making a total of 25 remedies for our differential diagnosis.

How do we justify the practice of allowing ourselves to be guided by mental symptoms in the selection of medicines for physical illness? Our experience has shown that "mentals" are often of overruling importance in determining the remedy which represents the total symptom complex similar to the patient's condition. Besides justifying our method of remedy selection, this fact also suggests that the mental attitudes, probably, are also of paramount importance in the establishment of the very psychosomatic complex itself, which represents the illness. By studying, in addition to abnormal chemistry, the mental attitudes of sick people, we may gain a deeper insight into the functioning of pathological happenings.

The provings, experimentally, demonstrate the fact that every constitutional brings forth mental symptoms. On the other hand, modern psychosomatic research has conclusively shown that mental and emotional attitudes deeply influence the physiologic functioning.

Thus, impatience, the symptom slated for our discussion, has to be looked upon as the expression of disturbed somatic functions as well as a factor which itself may call forth somatic pathology. The therapeutic requirement of the first premise leads to the differentiation of remedies by means of their mental symptoms; the second aspect calls for the task of inner self-development and of psychotherapy. Only to the extent that we keep sight of both of these sides will we be good physicians, not only good prescribers.

On the physical level, a cure can be accomplished only when the disease manifestation is not suppressed by *contrariis,* but is confronted with the similar, namely analogous, exogenous energy complex. In strict analogy, also on the psychological level, suppression by *contrariis* will not bring about a cure. Specifically, in the example of impatience, the contraria approach of mere rigid self-discipline or autosuggestion will succeed only in driving the disturbance underground. The psychological simile approach consists in the conscious confrontation with the conflicting elements of the unconscious, leading to a gradual understanding and conscious integration into a widened and deepened personality. The technique of this approach has been evolved, beyond the one-sided narrowness of Freud's approach, by the school of Analytical Psychology of Carl G. Jung.

Our meeting being concerned with the homeopathic tool, it is the first-mentioned task of differentiating the remedies characterized by impatience which commands our attention.

The symptom is of practical use for prescribing when it is found in a relatively outstanding degree; then it may be assumed to hold a key position in the total disorder. As long as a certain trait is relatively balanced and integrated into the total functioning, it is not pathogenetic. To some extent, everybody is impatient or indolent, irritable or fearful, etc. Consequently for the purpose of remedy selection, the symptom is of value only when it is:

1. One-sidedly outstanding in quantity (intensity), as in an excessively impatient person or in a quiet person who, contrary to his usual disposition, is acutely seized by his impatience,

2. When the symptom is a distinguishing factor by virtue, not of its quantitative, but of its qualitative importance. A person may not be excessively impatient but his impatience may still be quite characteristic and peculiarly distinctive for his very personality.

In case 1. we have to choose from among the comparatively acute remedies with strong impatience *(Acon., Ars., Bry., Cham., Coloc., Ign., Lach., Nux v., Rhus tox.)*, as well as from among those, of a more constitutional range, which have the symptom to an outstanding degree *(Ars., Hep., Ign., Iod., Lach., Med., Nux v., Sep., Sulf.)*.

In the more qualitative evaluation of case 2, we deal with broader constitutional types, impatience being but one qualifying symptom *(Arg. nit., Ars., Aur., Cal., Hep., Ign., Iod., Kali c., Lach., Lyc., Med., Nat. mur., Nux vom., Plat., Psor., Puls., Sep., Sil., Staph., Sulf.)*.

It must be borne in mind, however, that for didactic purposes we are drawing a line of division where in reality there are but fluid transitions. Therefore the division of remedies into acute and chronic should never become a rigid concept.

In our differential diagnosis, this time, we shall, expressly and deliberately, limit outselves to an investigation of the various types of impatience as they grow out of the overall psychological make-up of the patient. For reasons of time and space, only the main, pertinent points can be given; we shall disregard all other symptoms which, needless to say, must be considered in the actual, clinical remedy selection. This specialized study of a narrow field is offered as an addition and not instead of a thorough study of the broad remedy totality.

An evaluation of the psychological personality should be a part of the routine case taking. Particularly, when there is a dearth of sufficient generalities and modalities on which to base a proper prescription we can make the most of our evaluation of the psychological type.

ACONITE.

In the patient who requires *Acon.* the impatience springs from a state of panicky fear or fright. He vehemently and impatiently pleads that something be done to ward off the catastrophe which he feels to be impending. Though usually indicated in very acute states, it should not be forgotten in chronic states that developed after fright or shock.

ARSENICUM.

Also whenever *Ars.* is indicated the impatience stems from an underlying anxiety, be it conscious or unconscious. The *Ars.* personality is overexacting, overcritical and oversensitive, mercilessly and incessantly driving himself and those around him: quite aptly, this personality type has been likened to a racehorse. Whereas the anxiety of *Aconite* is associated with the violent assault of acutest congestion upon a hypersthenic type, the *Arsenicum* state may be described, more aptly, as irritable weakness with anguished restlessness, ending in extremes of prostration, more often found in the asthenic type.

RHUS TOXICODENDRON.

Rhus tox. has impatience springing also from irritable restlessness. Whereas *Ars.* is almost obsessed and driven mad by his restlessness, the *Rhus tox.* state is one of a more passive, yielding apprehension and impatience. In a picture that is shown by the fact that the *Ars.* patient is driven to shift from bed to bed or room to room, whereas the *Rhus* patient rolls and tosses, yet remains in bed.

CHAMOMILLA.

Cham. is in a state of frenzy, oversensitive to discomfort or pain, unable to endure anything or anybody and to control his or her uncivil temper. Nothing moves fast enough, nothing is being done properly, everything is rejected as soon as it has been carried out, according to the rapidly changing, capricious whims of the patient.

COLOCYTHIS.

Mentally, *Coloc.* is already over the worst and by the time you see him, he has calmed down and is suffering the physical consequences of his anger. Whereas *Cham.* may show you the door at your mere approach, *Colocynthis'* temper is hidden; he will not reveal it until you question him about it. His impatience springs from anger and vexation.

NUX VOMICA.

The impatience of *Nux vom.* may be less acute; however, it is rather deepseated, habitual and permanent. The *Nux* type is our well-known contemporary, the overcivilized city dweller, overintellectual or mentally overwrought, an overworked lawyer or bookkeeper, a tyrannical clerk, precise, fussy, critical, overbearing, oversensitive, jumpy and subject to fits of uncontrollable temper.

BRYONIA.

When anger, irritability and impatience do not find their expression in open outbursts, but keep slowly nagging and boring from within or remain completely unconscious, the rigid, tensive state of *Bryonia* develops. Like a bear chewing his paws, he wants to be left alone; he growls and snarls when you attempt to disturb him. Whereas *Nux vom.* is a more refined, even over-refined type, indulging in, and made ill, by mental intricacies as well as culinary delicacies, *Bry.* tends to be a more prosaic species concerned about business, stockmarket and daily bread; he is concerned with quantity rather than with quality. Thus, his suffering comes from business vexation and overeating.

Starting with "acute" medicines, we gradually are led to describe the broader constitutional states in the medicines that are to follow.

IGNATIA.

Ignatia's impatience springs from an emotional confusion. She is caught in an impasse of contradictory emotions or of emotions that conflict with the demands of reality. Usually refined, well-educated and cultured people, of a gentle disposition, the *Ignatia* patients are overwhelmed by emotional storms, grief over the loss of a dear person, or disappointment in love. Overwrought, aggrieved, lovelorn and lovesick, they are liable to strange actions and passionate outbursts. Their impatience, springing out of this overwrought almost hysterical state, is the expression of the desperate attempts to break free from the net in which they feel themselves entangled.

LACHESIS.

In *Lachesis,* the general keynote is suppression, physical, mental and emotional. Deepest passion, when denied open expression, is subject to perversion and turns into the venom of hatred, cruelty and jealousy. Suppressed unconscious emotions, like evil spirits continuously boring from within, permit no peace or quietness, resulting in *Lachesis'* restlessness, impatience, suspicion and anxiety.

SEPIA.

Whereas *Lachesis* is characterized by suppression in general, *Sepia* tends, more specifically, towards the frustration or inhibition of the feminine qualities. The *Sepia* patients are strongly emotional, yet repressed in their affections and their sexuality. The picture of love perverted into anger, spite, jealousy and hate, with the accompanying

181

restlessness and impatience, is quite similar to *Lach.,* therefore. However, in *Lach.* the perverted instinct tends to assume a ruthless permanent rule; in *Sepia,* the feminine quality, obscured and frustrated as it is, still, somehow and somewhere, manages to keep a woman gentle and yielding, as much as she may resent and try to hide this fact.

MEDORRHINUM.

The mental state of *Medorrh.* we might describe as being helplessly ridden by an unconscious panic. It appears as though a protective function of the inner life had broken down, allowing the patient to become a helpless prey of waves of anxiety, restlessness and hurried impatience. The mental powers may gradually fail, while the uncontrollable restless anguish, alternating with excessive languor and exhaustion, may take on an almost obsessive character.

ARGENTUM NITRICUM.

Arg. nitr., quite similarly, is a person ridden by anxiety, hurry and worry. However, whereas the mental state of *Medorrh.,* the nosode, appears to take effect by stunting and paralyzing the vitality, silver, the metal, affects the nervous functions primarily. Both, *Medorrh,* and *Arg. nitr.,* have the symptom of anticipation. *Medorrh,* with deeply disorganized vital, organic functions, shows a changed threshhold of consciousness, which anticipates, often correctly, unknown future events. *Argent. nitr.* is represented by the type of the overwrought, over-nerved intellectual worker or the neurotic, oversensitive, worn out and played out actor, who, panic-striken within, finds excuses for all of his shortcomings. He has exhausted his, however, normal mental functions and has lost his self-confidence. His anticipation is towards known and expected, rather than unknown, events. True to the neurotic pattern, this anticipation is transformed into physical symptoms.

IODUM.

Another personality, driven by restlessness and impatience, we meet in *Iodine.* Here, the restlessness strikes us as of a rather motor type. Constantly he must be active and on the move; he cannot sit still. Even his anxiety tends to take the form of fear of some imminent disaster, which demands some form of action. This motor restlessness, in which the patient literally burns himself up, we easily recognize as a manifest or occult hyperthyroidism.

SULPHUR

Sulphur, the king of the antipsorics, also is constantly on the go and bursting with initiative. The alchemists called *Sulphur* the "creator of a thousand things," the "heat and force of everything" and the "ferment which gives life, intelligence and colour to the imperfect bodies." Thus, the *Sulphur* personality, acting as a catalyst, always feels he must keep things and people on the move; he must always take the initiative, lest things become stagnant. He is ever full of new, often quite brilliant ideas, yet rather poor as to systematic planning and execution. *Sulphur* is impatient with those around him, with the slow world that cannot keep up with the speed and flight of his imagination. For every problem he quickly has a suggesion of what ought to be done, though, alas, it is not for him to waste his precious time in doing it; yet, the ungrateful world, never sufficiently seems to appreciate his genius. Could he be anything but impatient?

PSORINUM.

Comparable to a *Sulphur* state with a negative denominator, the antipsoric nosode has *Sulphur's* drive, but is utterly devoid of any vital energy to back it up. There is the same driving, impatient restlessness, but the optimistic sense of attainment is lacking. Instead of enthusiastically pushing on, *Psor.,* restlessly, keeps busy. Full of pessimism, gloom and despair, he expects to fail in every undertaking and to end up in the poorhouse.

HEPAR.

In *Hepar,* the *Sulphur* fire is modified by the *Calcarea* stagnancy and defenselessness. A peculiar state of hypersensitive, irritable sluggishness results, which is punctured by volcano-like eruptions of ire and wrath. *Hepar's* impatience bears the character of rashness and violence, of outbreaks of temper, of a person who cannot stand any opposition, unpleasantness or pain.

In the following group of medicines the impatience is likely to be more of a qualifying factor than quantitatively outstanding in intensity.

CALCAREA CARBONIA.

The typical *Calc.* patient may be likened to an oyster without a shell; he represents a helpless, flabby organism, lacking in inner organization and outer defense. He is easily exhausted, weak, sluggish and indifferent, lacks initiative, is unable to apply himself to any task and incapable of mental concentration. This weakness and helplessness breeds anxiety and worried, impatient nervousness.

SILICEA.

Comparing it to *Calcarea's* lack of a protective shell and inner organization, we may describe *Silicea* as rather well-organized, but devoid of fibre, stalk or firmness *(Sil.* is the main mineral constituent of stalks and fibrous tissues). Thus, *Sil.* tends to be a very orderly type of person, spic and span, but shy and timid without self-confidence, often anticipating failure. They are irritable and impatient when they are too hard pressed, aroused, or provoked.

PULSATILLA.
When we find the lack of stamina, not in the deepest grains of the personality, but rather in the more superficial form of emotional shiftiness and instability, the windflower, *Pulsatilla,* often the acute of *Sil.,* may be indicated. They are fickle, irresolute, impressionable, rather superficial types, always in need of emotional support and sympathy. Their mental and physical states are subject to frequent quick changes, forth and back, from complacent sweetness to irritable, fidgety impatience.

KALI CARBONICUM.
Kali carb. represents a changeable instability, often mindful of *Pulsatilla's* mental state. The *Kali carb.* condition seems part of a general state of low vital energy with disturbed adrenal functioning and vagotonia. The patient is whimsical, contradictory, quarrelsome, fearful and anxious. He is impatient, since his changing whims cannot be instantly heeded.

LYCOPODIUM.
Lycop. presents the trend of an intellectual overbalance, out of proportion to and at the expense of, an atrophying emotional life and of the purely vital energies. These patients are quite introverted, often asocial types; outwardly, perhaps, haughty and domineering, inwardly unsure of themselves, full of fears and feelings of inferiority. Irritability and impatience are the expressions of this precarious imbalance of their inner lives.

NATRUM MURIATICUM.
Also, the *Nat. nur.* patients are exceedingly introverted like the former, *Lycop.,* but their imbalance stems from a hypertrophy of emotion rather than of intellect. Their state is one of emotional isolation, be it self-imposed, or through the force of circumstances, such as bereavement and grief; violently and impatiently they resent any intrusion into the circle of their lonely withdrawal and introversion.

AURUM.
The gold patient, also, is lonesome and depressed. He is weighted down by a load of real or imagined responsibility, self imposed, or ordained by the necessity of circumstances. Thus, he is given to self accusations, brooding, melancholic depression, hopeless pessimism

and restless, impatient anxiety.

PLATINA.

Whereas *Aurum* tends to disparage and humble his ego, in relation to what he feels he should have attained, *Platina* aggrandizes himself and belittles his environment. He indulges in an assumed superiority of his self and disregards all that does not fit into the pattern of his self-inflation. For the sake of the power drive, the life of the other emotions and instincts is sacrificed and suppressed. A perverted instinctual and sexual life results, with irritability and impatience often of a definitely hysterical character.

STAPHISAGRIA.

Also *Staphisagria* tends to overrate his own importance, though often quite unaware of doing so. He is quite self-indulgent and will not deny himself the satisfaction of his emotional and sexual urges. Since he is very sensitive to the way he is judged, in relation to his own artificially maintained appearance, he easily lays himself open to injury to his pride, which, again, never must be admitted or noticed by others. The price for the maintenance of this artificial structure is paid for in tension, hysteria, spasticity and impatient irritability.

SURGERY: AN ATTITUDE OF PRESENT DAY MEDICINE

Within the last hundred years surgery has made rapid strides. From the most neglected it has developed into the most highly evolved branch of medicine. To a great extent public opinion identifies the successful doctor with the surgeon. And this growing esteem for surgery reveals an attitude of mind characteristic of our period.

Surgery, today, is used not only to correct damage resulting from injury, but, to an ever increasing extent, in the treatment of illness. But note that there is a fundamental difference between these two fields of application. The consequences of injuries are mechanical derangements of parts of a *healthy* organism, and it is obvious that for the correction of such conditions mechanical means are necessary. Surgery here is constructive.

It is different with disease. Here the disturbance is not of a mechanical nature and not caused from outside. Infection has been from time to time considered of outside origin, but sufficient evidence has accumulated to prove that it depends entirely upon the body's "resistance" whether or not an infection takes hold. An individual with no "disposition" for an infection may be exposed to pathogenic bacteria without suffering damage. Numerous doctors and nurses pass through epidemics unscathed. When an infection has already taken place, experience has demonstrated frequently that one can combat it more successfully, regardless of antibacterial measures, by strengthening the repelling and recuperative powers of the body. An organism in perfect balance of health lives in the constant presence of most of our pathogenic microorganisms without being affected. Only a derangement from within opens it to the infection.

The general explanation for the usefulness of surgery in the treatment of illness is that the human organism is a very complicated mechano-chemical machine. Each organ is compared to a part of a machine. Sickness is considered the failure of any of these parts to function properly, due either to outside damage or inner wear and tear. In a machine, damaged parts must be removed or exchanged. This solution is imitated by surgical removal and substitution therapy.

Certain processes within the human organism admit of purely mechanical and chemical explanations. Many processes in the living human body, on the other hand, act contrary to the chemical and mechanical laws of lifeless nature. When the severed (dismembered) ear of a rabbit is immersed in a mixture of pepsin and hydrochloric acid such as is found in the stomach, it is promptly dissolved and digested. When the unsevered ear of the living animal is dipped into the same mixture, nothing happens to it. The living organism voids and annuls the chemical attack.

One can study reactions which take place strictly and exclusively in accordance with the laws of outer chemistry in organs which have been removed from the body and are therefore in the process of disintegration, or when the whole organism has died. Then the mechanical and chemical forces of outer nature bring about the body's decomposition and disintegration. The life activities of the human body, on the other hand, tend to void, even actively oppose the chemical and mechanical laws of outer nature. No machine is gifted with life or can produce life. On the other hand, some life-inimical forces must be active to a certain extent, also within ourselves, bringing about the slow disintegration which is part of old age and leads to death.

Intimate observation shows that everything which has to do with feeling and consciousness tends to promote these processes of disintegration. One reason we feel refreshed and strengthened after sleep is that the destructive forces of consciousness are not active during sleep and a regeneration can be carried out by the opposite pole of vitality. On the other hand, without these decomposing forces of consciousness, man would always be asleep and not a full human being.

In our organism there is a polarity between the steady disintegration which follows and expresses the law of outer chemistry and the upbuilding forces of life and reproduction. The balance between these two extremes represents health. Any disturbance of the delicate balance between these two poles interferes with health. The vital forces can be weakened by improper living, dietary habits, climactic effects, and so forth. Disease will also be produced when the processes of decomposition are increased by influences from the soul life. Worry, sorrow or high tension, fear and hate, or even the inner difficulties of a developing personality, can produce sickness.

These factors, once understood, make it obvious that the abnormal structural changes found in diseased organs are consequences rather than causes of disturbance. They are end products of a metamorphosis which begins with changes in function and only gradually results in changes of chemistry and organic structure.

What then is the effect of the surgical removal of an abnormal part? Obviously it removes neither the cause of the disease nor the disease itself but does away only with the disease's result. To the extent that this has in itself become a source of disturbance to other parts, some immediate relief may follow surgery, and, indeed, if the disturbance has become dangerous, the life of the patient may be at least temporarily saved. Yet the basic disorder remains. If nothing is done by other methods to eradicate it, this basic disorder may progress toward new and greater destruction.

Its onward course seems to follow certain definite rules which are the reverse of Hering's Law of Cure. Any disorder first affects the less vital organs, the skin and peripheral parts. One gains the impression at times that the pathological state is trying to create an outlet for its waste products by maintaining an inflammation or continuous discharge from a bodily opening. When deprived of this primary expression by surgical removal or local treatment, the still existing basic condition has to move on to a new place of manifestation. The less vital part having been removed, a more vital organ will be affected next. When the peripheral lesion is closed, a disorder deeper inside starts. Whoever sees in disease only an isolated disturbance of a part of the "machine" fails to note these connections. Frequently a new condition is assumed and diagnosed when an old one is simply manifesting in a more insidious form. Another feat of surgery may then be recommended, and a vicious circle which can only lead to more and more destruction is created.

Even if one disregards the possible progress of an illness to more vital parts, the removal of an organ should not be looked upon too lightly. From the way this subject is generally discussed, one gains an impression that some organs in our body have no function whatsoever and had better be cut out as soon as possible — the appendix and tonsils, for instance.

But is an organ ever unnecessary? Is not the idea in itself absurd? Looking at nature and the cosmos, we can find only awe-inspiring greatness and the profoundest wisdom in every part of its creation. There are many things which we do not yet understand, but every new discovery serves to prove again this all-embracing wisdom. It is with an attitude of humility therefore, that a student of nature should approach unknown phenomena; and one cannot help feeling that it is a supercilious attitude lightly to declare, just because our restricted means of testing cannot explain its function, that a part of this most complicated, wisest member of all creation, the human organization, is unnecessary. It is characteristic of the present attitude of our science to assume the unimportance and inconsequence of what does not readily reveal its secret to our mechanistic methods. There is little willingness to trace events and effects which reveal themselves only to a more subtle observation.

No removal of an organ can be without disturbing consequences. The consequences may occur many years later and manifest as disturbances in quite remote regions and of a nature apparently unrelated to the original condition. It requires the most patient, the finest, really an almost artistic method of observation, to connect apparently unrelated phases of one and the same disturbance. And it is just this attitude of reverence, this ability to observe the human organization as the greatest work of art in the whole of creation, that is most lacking in the scientific research of our time.

All of this may appear a complete condemnation of surgery as applied to disease. It must be stressed therefore that surgery does have its place in the treatment of disease. Besides being indicated when a diseased part is disturbing other parts (as already discussed), it is frequently necessary for the purpose of creating an opening through which pus may be discharged. Furthermore it is justified when there is no other recourse left whatsoever, when the destruction has progressed so far that repair is impossible or when an urgently dangerous condition is present. But one should then consider surgery, by its very nature, not as a means of curing disease but as a necessary help in prolonging the life of the patient when a disease has become incurable.

It is interesting to note that, whereas today we tend to identify the successful doctor with the surgeon, in times past a distinction was made between the doctor who was to treat disease and the surgeon who was to remove the incurable. The use, even today, of the title "Physician and Surgeon" points to the fact that there must have once been a clear distinction. In contrast to our present attitude, surgery was not very highly respected in former times, and consequently was less highly developed than medicine. Today it is generally held that this low development of surgery was due to the fact that, anesthesia being for a long time unknown, certain major operations were out of the question. This, however, is not the case. Anesthetic and sleep-inducing drugs were known even in ancient times and, in one way or another, anesthesia was induced, though not as frequently and not with our present high degree of perfection. A student of medieval and, more particularly, of ancient medicine is rather tempted to wonder if the lack of skill in anesthetizing and surgery was not due to the fact that the doctors and priest healers of those times were indifferent to perfecting them inasmuch as they felt that their real task was to cure with the forces from within rather than to mutilate. Hippocrates the "father of medicine" was the last important disciple of the ancient priestly healing centers who apparently possessed a vast instinctive insight into the curative powers of herbs, minerals and metals. However, beyond this instinctive approach there was not yet any real scientific understanding. During the following centuries a thoughtless traditionalism took rule in medicine. An ever increasing confusion and irrational abuse of drugs and poisons reached its climax during the 17th and 18th centuries. The scientific method of research ushered in a new era of natural science which set out to dispose of this intolerable chaos. Towards this end Samuel Hahnemann proceeded by his exact method of testing each single drug on healthy human individuals and for the first time in the history of mankind experimentally established the exact relationship between each drug and the diseased state which it can cure. This relationship is summarized in the "law of similars" which forms the basis of Homeopathy. However, the majority of doctors, up to the very present, refuse even to investigate Hahnemann's discoveries and limit their experiments instead to animals and isolated, cut-out organs. They lose sight of the fact that a living human organism, the carrier of a conscious personality, is an inseparable whole and differs from an isolated organ, which is in a state of decomposition or from a test animal which has an entirely different soul-body structure. In comparison to the homeopathic experiment on human provers, the animal experiment is inexact and unreliable. It divulges only the crudest toxic properties of medicinal substances warranting their use for the suppression of single symptoms only, but not for a harmonious cure of the whole psychosomatic soul-body disturbance which lies at the bottom of all illness.

Modern allopathic medicine excels in diagnostic casuistry — and leads to therapeutic nihilism. No wonder that the surgeon triumphantly conquered the field from which the physician had resigned. Is there any hope that some day medicine may again become a science and art of real healing rather than of mutilation? Only a recognition of the necessity of patiently observing what is behind purely mechanical and chemical happenings can meet this challenge. Homeopathy has developed the scientifically exact experimental method which initiates such a new understanding for man as the integrated unit of body, soul and spirit — a real fulfillment of psychosomatic medicine. It is up to the coming generations to forego again the limelight of the operating room for the quiet work of the patient healer.

Part IV
CASE STUDIES

ALLERGIC DIATHESIS

The two cases presented here have been chosen for the fact that their curative remedies are relatively less known and insufficiently proven, yet have a wide constitutional range of action.

The first is a four-year-old boy with recurrent serious attacks of bronchial asthma. Twice in the past he had to be hospitalized for status asthmaticus with bronchopneumonia. He is dark-complexioned and plump, pasty and pale with dry skin. He makes a slow, apathetic impression, is very easily tired but also easily irritated, very emotional and sensitive. The condition is worse in winter, worse from chocolate and particularly worse from milk, which is also disliked, and worse from damp weather. There is easy perspiration, especially of the hands and head.

For a while his condition improved under *Calcarea carbonica.* Then the asthmatic tendency recurred and failed to respond to repetitions and higher potencies of *Calcarea carbonica.*

Now the prescription was *Viscum album* 200. At the height of an acute asthma attack, *Viscum* proved the needed intercurrent. It controlled the acute exacerbations. *Calcarea carbonica* now again worked as a constitutional protection, gradually reducing the intensity of the onset of the attacks. The attacks themselves required *Viscum album.* The complementary use of *Calcarea* chronically and *Viscum* acutely gradually normalized the condition.

A translation of the *Viscum album* proving appeared in the May-June 1960 Journal of the American Institute of Homeopathy. I merely repeat here the most characteristic points of its symptomatology. *Viscum album* is a spastic drug fitted for nervous, emotional and spastic disturbances in a wide range of oversensitive individuals. The *Viscum* patient is sad, tired, feels worn out, is apathetic but restless at the same time, over-sensitive to noise, has an aversion to people, wants to be left alone, cannot react adequately to people. There is a tendency to go to extremes: over-stimulation, intense almost manic ability to react, as well as, more often, a depressive oversensitivity. Vertigo is a leading symptom. Along with the *Magnesias, Mandragora, Phosphorus* and *Conium maculatum, Viscum is one of the leading vertigo remedies.* Its symptoms are worse at night. It has a distinctive organ affinity in neuro-vegetative disturbances particularly relating to the circulatory and respiratory systems. It should be thought of first in *spastic cough* with dyspnoea and irritation, *bronchial asthma, angina pectoris,* coronary conditions, cardiac neuroses, cardiac disturbances of emotional origin such as paroxysmal tachycardia, and possibly any other functional or organic interference with cardiac innervation.

The second case is a girl of 16 who is allergic to lipstick. Whenever she used lipstick her lips would break out, the skin would crack and a rash appear around the lips. She also suffered from vasomotor rhinitis, conjunctival itching and irritation. This, however, did not bother her. The inability to use lipstick represented a personal tragedy.

She is thin, of almost transparent appearance, dark-complexioned with large eyes, very sensitive, excitable. There is a tendency to take colds easily. She is very chilly. She tends to be nauseated. There are menstrual cramps, and pains in the legs like "growing pains."

The remedy first prescribed was *Phosphorus*; it had a moderate effect but did not hold. It was followed by *Psorinum* with a similar poor effect. The case was now restudied and the prescription was *Thyroidin 200*, which in varying potencies proved the indicated remedy, covering adequately and successfully the symptomatology.

Let me review briefly the symptomatology of *Thyroidin* which, though inadequately known, is a constitutional remedy of the widest range when used in potency.

Thyroidin patients are chilly; only rarely are they warm-blooded. They are of thin builds, of nervous temperaments, and with prominent eyes. The remedy is not contraindicated for fat persons, however. The *Thyroidin* patient has puffiness of the face and a tendency to angioneurotic edema, urticaria, asthma and eczema. In other words, *Thyroidin* in potency covers the allergic, angio-neurotic and vasomotor constitution in its various manifestations. People needing *Thyroidin* are nervously and emotionally affected showing disturbances of the vasomotor balance, hysterical and allergic tendencies.

It fits convulsions of the new born, vomiting of babies after birth (sometimes with jaundice), the vomiting and diarrhea of dentition, and infantile marasmus. It is indicated for the results of over-indulgence in sexual activity, for the effects of disturbed sexual function, for complaints incidental to and aggravated by menstrual disturbances or irregularity. Thus, it suits the symptoms of puberty as well as of the menopause, the mental disturbances of puberty and menopause and those following childbirth.

In the above conditions, when the apparently indicated familiar remedy fails, *Thyroidin* may be called for. It is the nosode for the allergically, hysterically and emotionally disturbed vasomotor constitution.

NEW OR FORGOTTEN INDICATIONS
OF TUBERCULIN

S.B., age 3. Purulent bilateral otitis media. In spite of a continuous discharge from both ears, continuing pain and 101° to 103° fever. Better from hot applications; the discharge is yellow and sticky. The child is light-complexioned, blond and chubby; constitutionally, there is poor appetite, a tendency to constipation and considerable perspiration of the head. Tendency to repeated high fevers. For the last six months prior to the onset of the present illness this child had made general progress under Calcarea carbonica 200 to 1 M; yet, the present condition has arisen in spite of a recent repetition of Calcarea. Rx: Hepar sulphuris 200; no response. Sulfur, Silica, and Pulsatilla (in disregard of the local modality) also failed. An otological consultant urges Penicillin in oil 300,000 Units; this is given without any appreciable effect. Now Bacillinum 30 a single dose is given. There is a sharp rise of the temperature which subsides after a few hours. Within 24 hours the temperature drops to normal and the pain disappears. Two days later no more discharge from the ear and eventual recovery.

Mr. E.S., age 41, a hairdresser by occupation. Chronic eczema of both hands, groins and feet. Patch-tests have furnished conclusive evidence that the condition is due to an allergy to the hairdyes which he has to use in his work. Whenever he stops using the hairdyes his skin clears up. Upon resumption of the work the eczema returns. Since he owns his small business he must continue to work. He wishes to be freed of his oversensitivity. The skin specialists and allergists he has consulted before have assured him that this is impossible. Constitutionally, he is thin, narrow-chested, of a sallow complexion and a sanguine temperament, restless, jumpy, irritable and impatient. He perspires freely and is disturbed by his own body odor. Sensitive to drafts of air with a tendency to frequent colds and generally feeling worse in winter; hot burning feet which he likes to uncover. Tendency to constipation, desire for meat and highly seasoned foods. Obviously, this is a clear case for Sulfur. Yet, alas, Sulfur makes no impression at all upon this patient.

When the apparently well indicated remedy fails we are taught to prescribe Sulfur. What, however, should be our prescription when as in this case, Sulfur itself is the apparently well selected remedy? On the basis of the therapeutic rule, outlined at the end of this paper, Tuberculin is given. The apparently impossible task is accomplished for this patient. Several doses of Tuberculin restore him to fairly normal skin, in spite of his continued use of his hairdyes.

Mr. W. G., age 47. History of repeated severe gallbladder attacks. Being extremely weakened by the frequently occuring colics, cholecystectomy has been advised. The attacks shown no characteristic or unusual symptoms. He is a laborer, short, stout, of stocky square build and somewhat slow in his response and reactions. Easily perspiring, fond of sweets, constipated but with too excellent an appetite, he often gets his attacks after overeating. Rx: Calcarea carbonica ranging from 200 to 10M over a year. During this period there is a considerable improvement, generally, as well as in the frequency and intensity of his attacks, which finally do not occur any more at all. However, a considerable amount of abdominal discomfort continues to annoy him. Also, some new symptoms, in the form of pains in the right elbow and the lower back, stubbornly persist. Again, Tuberculin is prescribed, with a resulting complete removal of the totality of the gallbladder as well as rheumatic symptoms.

We have discussed a case, of each acute otitis media, chronic eczema, and cholecystopathy. Not in any of these clinical conditions would we, as a rule, think of Tuberculin, in spite of the fact that Allen's Nosode list: "discharge of yellowish matter from ears, swelling of glands around ears, cramping pains in stomach and abdomen, colic with great thirst, pain achin sticking in region of the liver, bloated sensation in abdomen, eczema, itching burning oozing, forming scabs." Unfortunately, we are in the habit of thinking of Tuberculin as a remedy limited to the various ailments of the phthisical type of constitution and to chest conditions in particular. In my own experience Tuberculin has proven to be a polychrest of the first order which, on the average, is indicated as often as Sepia, Nux Vomica, Phosphorus, Pulsatilla, etc. It may be considered second only to Sulfur in the frequency of requirement. Since, like Sulfur, its pathogenetic sphere seems to cover almost any ailment to which man is heir, we cannot prescribe it primarily on clinical considerations any more than for instance Sulfur or Sepia. Conditions as divergent, clinically, as arthritis, hayfever, cystitis, pyelitis, hemorrhoids, cholecystopathy, chronic dyspepsia, pneumonia, thyroid disorders, otitis media, sciatica, migraine, eczema have been cured by its prescription. Quite obviously, a successful prescription has to be based upon the mentals and generals for this remedy not any less than for any of the other polychrests. The difficulty of applying this rule to Tuberculin lies in the fact that Kent's as well as Boeninghausen's *Repertory* take, at best, only very scanty notice of it and, on the other hand, no single, individual materia medica presents a fully exhaustive, comprehensive account of the totality of its symptoms. Though, Clarke's *Dictionary* might be considered to come the closest to a comprehensive picture of our remedy it still is highly advisable to study it from several different sources. If we were to give a general characterization in the form of a single therapeutic rule we might state that in addition to the symptoms already listed in the Materia Media, it also partakes in the symptomatology not only of Phosphorus but almost even more so, of Sulfur and Calcarea carbonica.

It should be axiomatic to consider Tuberculin the nearest complementry remedy to Sulfur, Calcarea, and Phosphor. As a safe therapeutic rule, not for automatic prescribing, of course, but rather for the priority of remedy study in a given case, we may establish that any case which presents the symptom picture of Sulfur, Calcarea, or Phosphor, yet fails to respond to the apparently well chosen remedy is to be considered a case for Tuberculin.

When we encounter a patient who fails to respond to the apparently well indicated remedy we consider his lack of reaction an expression of "psora", according to Hahnemannian precepts. We now search for an "antipsoric" prescription, from among such remedies as Calcarea, Lycopodium, Sulphur, Carbo vegetabilis, etc. Yet what are we to do about a case that by its symptoms, from the very onset, clearly demands Sulphur, Calcarea, Lycopodium, or any other of those medicines listed by Hahnemann as antipsoric and yet just as clearly, fails to respond to them. It is postulated that such a situation demands the prescription of a nosode. Regardless of whether or not we believe in Hahnemann's theory of miasms (the best theories are but temporary rationalizations of enigmatic facts), empirically we know that there exists a complementary relationship of remedies; this knowledge enables us to select a second and third prescription capable of correcting the failure of the first apparently well indicated remedy. Purely empirically, to give some simple examples, there are complementary group relations between Mercury, Hepar sulphuris and Silica; Mercury, Aurum, Kali iodatum, and Nitric acid; Arsenicum album, Lachesis, Lycopodium, and Hepar sulphuris. All of these in turn are related complementarily to Syphilinum.

Sepia, Thuja, Staphisagria, Nitric acid, and Argentum nitricum again are related to each other as well as to Medorrhinum.

Calcarea, Sulphur, Lycopodium, Magnesium, Sepia, Phosphorus, Kali carbonicum, Carbo vegetabilis, Graphites, Nitric acid, Causticum, etc. represent a family related to Tuberculinum, Psorinum, Streptococcin and to the intestinal nosodes.

Mr. H. S., age 50. For the last ten years complaining of gas and abdominal distention, slight tendency to constipation, lack of appetite, swollen gums, mouth odor, etc. He has resorted to vegetarianism and is a thorough hypochondriac in the most literal meaning of the word. Eccentric ideas, lanky thin, stooping, skin slightly unclean. Gastro-intestinal examination is clinically and roentgenologically negative. Sulphur gives but temporary relief. Finally, after almost losing one's faith in the ability to help him, Morgan pure 200 does the trick. Now the improvement is permanent, necessitating one prescription but once a year.

Mr. A. N., age 50. Old recurring otitis media right ear with offensive discharge. Tendency to headcolds, congestive occipital headaches with vomiting, worse from smell of foods. Very much intestinal fermentation and distention. Pressure and fullness in the liver area, anal itching. History of small rightsided kidney stones. Tendency to lumbago. He craves sweets, is sensitive to tight clothing, chilly but better in the open air and better from motion. The symptoms definitely seem to point to

Lycopodium. Actually Lycopodium always gives prompt relief but in spite of trying the whole range of potencies, fails to prevent a recurrence of his difficulties. Also here Morgan pure 200 turned out to be the true constitutional prescription covering both the acute as well as the chronic phases.

Mrs. H. H., age 29. For six years suffering from gallstone colics in ever increasing severity. Lost ten pounds of weight during the last six weeks. At present, pains in the gallbladder area start about 20 minutes after eating and radiate to the right shoulder. Very much abdominal distention with eructations. Constipation with laxative habit. The pains are better from hot applications and better after eructations. She desires sweets and fats which aggravate her symptoms. She is sensitive to pressure of clothes around the waist. The menses are late and scanty and she is worse before menstruation. Mentally introverted, of dark complexion, early graying of hair, irritable and impatient. Lycopodium in varying potencies gave a good response but no lasting improvement could be accomplished. Morgan Gaertner 200, 4 doses within 3 months changed the picture completely. For the last 1½ years the patient has been completely free from any disturbances.

Mrs. M. H., age 27. Was seen first five years ago presenting the prescriber with the problem of ever recurring colds, usually with fever. They start in the throat and end in the chest or nose. History of recent broncho-pneumonia. Very few individualizing symptoms are available. The patient is tall, heavy, fair complexioned, blond or rather pasty appearance, but mentally very active. Chilly, worse from dampness, worse in the winter, desire for sweets and highly seasoned food. The main remedies were Calcarea carbonica and Sulphur. After two years the severity of the colds had considerably decreased but the frequency of their occurrence was still the same. In view of the apparently insufficient response to the obviously indicated remedy a nosode seemed indicated; but neither Tuberculinum nor Psorinum seemed to be of any help. Then it was noted that frequently the beginning of a cold coincided with intensified halitosis and constipation. Through these however vague hints, the attention was drawn to the intestinal tract as a concomitant factor. Sycotic Co. 200 provided the constitutional answer to her problem and freed her from her liability to colds.

The keynote given by Paterson ("The Bowel Nosodes"; *The British Homoeopathic Journal,* July 1950) for Morgan (Bach) is "congestion." "Spasm" might be appropriately added. The medicine covers that range of functions and localizations which we commonly associate with Sulphur and Lycopodium. Its foremost localizations of action are the gastrointestinal system (congestive, spastic, biliary conditions), respiratory tract (bronchitis, pneumonia, particularly of children), skin (chronic eczemas), and head (congestive headaches). It is generally worse from heat, worse before thunderstorms, worse from riding trains or buses and worse from excitement. The personality type is marked by great introspection, anxiety about his health and depression. With Lycopodium it shares the peculiar symptom of aversion to company, yet fear when alone.

The sub-type Morgan Gaertner seems more likely indicated in the presence of actual cholecystitis (according to Paterson, also in nephro-lithiassis). In my own experience, the differentation of Morgan (Bach) and Morgan pure may be quite difficult at times without the aid of an objective method of remedy selection.

For Sycotic Co. Paterson gives "irritability" as keynote. Perhaps "oversensitiveness" should be added as a modifying description of the factor which conditions the irritability. Fear of the dark, of being alone, emotional repressions. The irritability also applies physically to mucous and synovial membranes. Typical constitutional features are pasty, waxy, anemic, or sallow complexions with oily skin. There is a pronounced exudative diathesia which expresses itself in all sorts of allergies, inflammations and "colds." The nearest resemblance is to Tuberculinum. Paterson also mentions Lycopodium, Thuja, and Nitric acid as related constitutional remedies but stresses the fact that Sycotic Co. is to be considered a pretuberculous medicine corresponding to a catarrhal tendency.

Hahneman's theory of chronic miasms is one of his most significant contributions to the management of chronic illness. Yet, given our present understanding of pathophysiology, it is also the most obscure. It has met with persistent opposition even among his followers, and with ridicule outside of homeopathy. According to Hahneman the origin of all chronic disorders resides in three "miasms"—Psora, Sycosis, and Syphilis. According to the dictionary, miasms are "noxious emanations of imponderable nature." Hahneman himself took the existence of such miasms for granted; they were in fact standard entities in eighteenth century medicine and did not require further definition anywhere during his lifetime.

Nowadays entities of this sort appear utterly vague and unscientific. We accept that two hundred years ago "nebulous miasms" may have been postulated for lack of more precise knowledge, but in our time definite microorganisms have been identified. Syphilis and gonorrhea, and the various "psoric" skin conditions (notably scabies), are caused not by "miasmatic" influences affecting the body's entire functioning but invasions of germs from local infections. Moreover, since in most chronic diseases no microorganisms, least of all syphilitic or gonorrheic ones, can be demonstrated, the assumption of syphilitic or gonorrheic origination is rather absurd in most unspecific disorders. The belief that miasms cause chronic diseases would not seem anymore promising initially than the belief that deleterious effects can originate in witchcraft or the evil eye.

The homeopathic practitioner may also wonder whether—in the absence of a gonorrheic, syphilitic, or dermatologic history—the psoric, syphilitic or sycotic origin of a chronic state simply can be deduced from the fact that the ailment satisfactorily responds to one of the so-called "antipsoric," "antisyphilitic," or "antisycotic" remedies. It is in view of this dilemma that we shall reevaluate and rethink the evidence concerning the chronic miasms.

Obviously a condition cured by a drug classified as antisycotic f.i. Thuja need not necessarily be gonorrheic, nor does a response to Mercury prove a syphilitic origin. However, when a chronic condition responds to a nosode like Medorrhinum or Syphilinum, there must be some connection between Gonorrhea or Syphilis and the patient's condition. It may therefore prove helpful to approach our problem from the vantage of the clinical evidence furnished by the action of these nosodes. We shall arbitararily choose Syphilinum as an example.

In its provings on the healthy individual, Syphilinum produces symptoms which can be classified in two groups. The first group (A) bears a definite resemblance to the symptoms of clinical syphilis in its various stages (chancroid ulcers, copper-colored eruptions, nightly bone pains, cephalalgia, etc.). In the second group (B) of typical Syphilinum symptoms (fear of night, loss of memory, craving for alcohol, ozaena, ulcers of tonsils, etc.) we can not yet see any convincing evidence of clinical syphilis.

Both of these groups of symptoms are produced by material which, because of its high attenuation in potency, cannot contain any spirochetes. Nor can one by any stretch of imagination classify the disturbance produced by the proving of the nosode as an "infection." Yet we cannot deny that in group A symptoms a syphilis-like picture arises from this non-material attenuation consisting not of spirochetes but constituting a dynamic energy, indeed an "emanation of imponderable nature." Here is experimental evidence of emanations much like those in the dictionary definition of "miasm"—emanations capable of causing disturbances of health. Here is not merely unscientific phantasy but demonstrable fact.

What is the nature of the pathological conditions thus produced? Having been called forth by potentized syphilitic material (which in this form meets the definition of the miasm), both group A and group B symptoms are expressions of the healthy prover of a syphilitic miasm. Furthermore we see that the sphere of action of this miasm includes (in its group A symptoms) but also surpasses (with group B) what we now define as clinical syphilis, i.e., the symptoms of a syphilitic infection.

When we encounter a patient who exhibits symptoms which in their totality resemble group A or group B or a combination of them, Syphilinum will be the curative remedy. The same would be true if his case showed a close resemblance to a totality of group B symptoms. Does that mean that we are justified in classifying his disorder as syphilitic in this latter case also even if there is no personal or familial history whatsoever of a clinical syphilitic infection? If Syphilinum cures, can one simply dismiss that fact by considering the state an entirely different, namely nonsyphilitic condition for which syphilinum just "happens" to be the remedy? What, after all, is the *functional significance* of the fundamental homeopathic formula, *similia similibus curentur*—"let likes be cured by likes?" Hahneman stated it as no more than a rule for practical therapeutics. He did not declare a natural law, nor did he concern himself with an explanation of dynamics which express themselves through similarity.

What really is the relation between the symptoms of the prover and of the similar illness? We cannot yet say with certainty that a remedy cures *because* it is capable of producing symptoms which are similar to the patient's. The *similia similibus* does not offer any explanation for the ability to cure; it explains only *when* a remedy will cure, not *why* it cures. This "why" touches upon the basic dynamics of analogy in nature; yet we have been at a loss for an explanation. In fact, we have avoided thinking about it. Physics, however, furnishes us with a phenomenon which may help our understanding, namely that of the interference of light or, generally, wave patterns. Two vibratory energies of *identical* nature—that is, identical vibratory rate and frequency but of opposite origin, direction or phase—abolish each other when they meet. This would seem the very phenomenon that we encounter when the vibratory energy of the potentized drug neutralizes the vibratory energy of the disease. Hence, by analogy with the example of physics, we may postulate that the drug energy must be of identical nature, i.e. vibratory rate and frequency, as the disease energy. Drug and disease differ only in phase, namely origin and direction. The energy of the remedy is of exogenous origin, a part of external nature; the disease originates within the patient. Like Paracelsus we should speak of a mercury, a syphilis-like, or a gold disease—the metals or nosodes in nature representing the similar disease within the patient. And we may accept the fact that any disorder exhibiting the Syphilinum symptoms and curable by this nosode must be the Syphilinum disease, i.e. the expression of the syphilitic miasm in the patient, even if there is no resemblance or history of what we commonly call clinical syphilis.

In defining the sphere of the syphilitic miasm in terms of the symptoms of the nosode and of related remedies, we find that what we once called syphilis in the clinical sense is but a small part of its whole miasmatic sphere. We often encounter the miasmatic symptoms in patients without clinical syphilis, but never do we find clinical syphilis without the miasmatic symptoms. Would this not justify the conclusion that the miasmatic state is a prior condition, and the clinical syphilis secondary, incidental to it? When a person is constitutionally affected by the syphilitic, sycotic, or psoric miasm, he may fall prey to an infection of spirochetes, gonocci, or any of the germs found in the psoric conditions. Exposure to a discrete source of infection results in a "taking" of the infection only in some, not in all individuals thus exposed. The discrepancy has been explained by a so far undefined resistance factor or by a highly hypothetical skin injury. We may feel justified in the assumption that this resistance depends at least partly upon the miasmatic predisposition.

It is not clinical syphilis, gonorrhea, or scabies then that underlie chronic diseases. Neither are they, as our present theories would have us believe, incidental and merely external local infections. They are rather expressions of specific preexisting disturbances of the patient's life energy. Any influence which engrafts or increases the miasmatic influence or is otherwise capable of converting the chronic state into an acute one will produce the picture of clinical syphilis, gonorrhea, or one of the psoric manifestations, thereby creating locally a suitable environment for the growth of germs which would be repelled in a non-miasmatic state. Perhaps, as our proving experiments have shown us, when the exogenous impact happens to be disproportionately strong or repetitive it can even engraft the miasmic field on an organism that under ordinary circumstances would not "take" to it. We see this phenomenon in epidemics and in the response to "epidemic remedies" which are reflections of the "current" miasm.

As yet we cannot define the nature of the miasms any better than by stating that they resemble an energy which in outer nature is represented by the dynamic forces of Syphilinum, Medorrhinum, Psorinum, Mercury, Thuja, Sulfur, etc., and that they also can be engrafted on a previously healthy organism in a manner not unlike a proving when the proving is extended beyond individual tolerance. The old definition of a miasm as a noxious emanation of imponderable nature still seems as good as any to appear since.

Once we admit that the symptoms of group A or B are the true expressions of the syphilitic miasm, we must apply this relationship to any other remedy producing and curing these symptoms. The similarity between the totality of the patient's and the prover's symptoms is not a superficial coincidence but the expression of the identity of the basic energies in both the remedy and the disease. We are entitled, therefore, to the conclusion that, to the extent that Syphilinum, Mercury, Aurum or other substances share symptoms recognized as syphilitic, they also share and express the syphilitic miasm.

Syphilis and Sycosis offer relatively simple drug and disease pictures by comparison to psora which Hahneman called the thousand-headed hydra. The principles discerned for syphilis and sycosis must, however, apply equally to psora, despite its multiple character.

The miasms may express themselves in acute peripheral manifestations on the skin, the genitals, etc. These cases, as we know, give the better prognosis. The more difficult cases of chronic diseases are those where the peripheral manifestations have been suppressed or where peripheral manifestations have never taken place: insidious psora, syphilis, and sycosis.

What are the miasms, really? In view of their analogy to the effects of the potentized drug and their capacity to be engrafted (note also that the remedy effect can be engrafted as well upon non-living substance, such as glass, cork and sugar granules), we might consider them structural or archetypal fields of force, vortices of energy. They are capable of destructuring living activity but must in one way or another also be integral life and consciousness enhancing factors of the human constitution. Their classification into only psora, syphilis, and sycosis appears insufficient to me. Tuberculosis and Carcinosis at least need to be added. With closer scrutiny we may find more. Indeed closer inquiry into the "personalities" of the miasms remains a challenging task of further research.

GENERAL INDEX

abstraction, defined, 119
Aconite, 28
adrenalin formation, 99
adrenal gland, 100; dysfunction of, 101, 111
Aesculapius, 131-132, 136
air hunger, 138
alchemy, 32-33, 51
___, analytic psychology and, 76
___, dreams and, 77
___, Jung and, 76
___, salt and, 86
allergic diathesis, 193-194
analogical thinking, 7
Anacardium Orientale, 28
analytic psychology, 24, 31, 41
anemia, 111
anesthetics, 112-115
anima, 97
animal testing, 190
animus, 97
antimony, 28
antipsorics, 77, 79
antisycotic drugs, 201
Archeus, 176
archetypal images, 8, 41
archetype, 53
Aristolochia, for labor and gangrene, 150
Arnica montana (leopard's bane), 176
arthritis (spinal), 22
"Arzneimittle Bilder" (remedies as personalities), 130-131

Bacchus, 110
Backster, Clive, 61
Belladona, 28
biological time, 168
Blake, William, 10
Boeninghausen's *Repertory*, 196
Boericke's *Materia Medica*, 140
breathing, breath control, 114
bronchial asthma, 193
Bryonia, 21

Calcarea carbonica (calcium carbonate), 119-129, 140, 170, 195-197, 198, 199
___, energy field and, 120
___, features common with *Magnesium*, 120
___, feminine principle and, 93
___, walling off and, 123
Calcarea Ostrearum (oyster shell), 26, 33
Calcium, 116, 120-129
Carrabis Indica, 170
Carbo Animalis, 137-140;
___, aging and, 137
Carbo vegetabilis (vegetable charcoal), 137-140, 198
Cartesian dichotomy, 9
Carcinosis, 204
causality and non-causality, 69
___, physics and, 69
___, potency and, 94
___, synchronicity and, 73
cause and effect, 16
Chardin, Pierre Teilhard de, 11, 64
choleric, 69
Christianity, 49
chronic prescribing, 164-172
chronic miasms *(Psora, Sycosis, Syphilis)*, 201-204
clairvoyance, 109
Clarke's *Dictionary*, 196
collective unconscious, 86
complementary balance, law of, 36
complementation (complementary evolution), 24
Conium maculatum (poison hemlock), 170
constitution, 44-48
Copernicus, 8
coryza, 20

daimonion (Socratic; autonomous spirit in nature), 49, 98
Darwin, 130
depth psychology, 7
diabetes, 114
dreams, use of, 46
drug pictures, 120
dualistic (medicine), 24, 31

Einsteinian revolution, 52
emotional suppression, 30
energy field, 16, 21, 160
___, chronic miasms and, 204
___, light and, 159

Salt *(Natrium Chloride)*, also *Sal*, 26, 40, 106-107
Saturn, 62
Schroedinger, E., 72, 74, 80
sciatica, 22
scientific method, 24
Sepia (ink of squid or cuttlefish), 56-59, 92-104, 151, 196
____, Calcerea, Phosphor and, 100
____, characteristics of mollusks and, 92
____, impatience and, 181
____, feminine principle and, 93
____, *Lachesis* and, 133
____, melanin and, 95
____, self-enclosed softness and, 93
shadow (Jung's conception of), 46
Silica, 195
Silicea, 183-184
similars, law of, 94, 202
simillimum, 9, 11, 43, 47, 140, 157, 176
sinnbilder (German image of meaning or symbol), 131
Sodium, 121
soul, 77
space-time, 52
spirochetes, 203
Staphisagria, 28, 185
Steiner, Rudolf, 106
Stearns, F., 170
stomach, 147
subatomic, 8
Sulfur (Sulphur), 40, 47, 74-80, 99, 140, 182-183, 195, 196, 198, 199
____, alchemy and, 76-77
____, personality type, 75-76
surgery, 186-190
Sycotic Co. (Sycosis), 200, 204
symbolic perception, 54
symbols, 46
symbolic thinking, 7, 41
synchronicity, 29
____, absolute knowledge and, 73
____, as category of scientific thinking, 73
____, depth psychology and, 71
syphilis, 166, 198, 201
Syphilinim (nosode), 201-204
Syphillitic miasm, 201-204

technology, 49
Theokritos, 49
Thuja, 198, 200, 201

Thyroiden, for allergic, 194
totality (symptom, patient, remedy), 165
Tuberculin, 195-197, 198, 204
tuberculosis, 115, 166

uncertainty principle, 69

vertigo, remedies for, 193

Wheeler, C.E., 64

Ying/Yang, 124

Zeus, 106